CALLAN PARK

HOSPITAL FOR THE INSANE

Sarah Luke is an English and History teacher based in Sydney. She enjoys writing fiction and non-fiction, and always with a strong nineteenth-century flavour. Sarah is a member of the Friends of Callan Park and finds old Australian institutions enduringly interesting. Her website is sarah-luke.com.

CALLAN PARK

HOSPITAL FOR THE INSANE

SARAH LUKE

Australian Scholarly

To my Dad,

and to my real and imagined friend,

Mr Legard, Esq

First published 2018 by
Australian Scholarly Publishing Pty Ltd
7 Lt Lothian St Nth, North Melbourne, Vic 3051
Tel: 03 9329 6963 / Fax: 03 9329 5452
enquiry@scholarly.info / www.scholarly.info

ISBN 978-1-925588-96-5

Cover design: Wayne Saunders
Cover photo: Mitchell Library, State Library New South Wales [PX*D 241].
Original source: 'Callan Park, A Great State Institution', *Sydney Mail,*
12 August 1903, photographs by Alfred Small

CONTENTS

APPENDICES

ACKNOWLEDGMENTS

This book would never have been published without the interest and care of Nick Walker and his team at Australian Scholarly Publishing. I cannot thank them enough.

The research and writing of this book has led me to many new places and people, each of whom has assisted this book to fruition. My special thanks to the Friends of Callan Park, who have adopted me as one of their own, and always supported and encouraged me in my research and publishing goals. Particular thanks go to Roslyn Burge, whose lively appreciation of my research I will always treasure.

My sincere gratitude goes to colleagues Jillian Anderson and Julie Wilson Reynolds, who originally sent me to Callan Park in 2015 for a course at the NSW Writers' Centre. I had never been to Callan Park before, and as I typed its name into Google Maps I had no idea that it would change my life so dramatically. Further thanks to Julie for sending me to London in 2016 where I could complete my research at the British Library and National Archives in person, and visit St Nicholas for myself. I will never forget the quietness and tranquillity of Ganton – and it was a privilege to walk in Mr Legard's holy shoes if only for a day.

Thank you, too, to all of the archivists and knowledgeable people who have assisted me with queries about 'lunatics who I am not actually related to'. First place must go to NSW State Records, where the staff are most amazing. Thank you also to Cassie Watson at the NSW Writers' Centre for her help with wallpaper and basements; the SCA for their open-door policy; Jenny Pearce at the King's School Archive; the staff at the Charterhouse School Archive and the East Riding Archive; the volunteers at the SPASM Museum, and all the other people who have helped out in small yet significant ways.

Thank you to Sue Stenning for advice and downloads. Thank you to Sue Corrigan who met me outside the Ganton Greyhound on a lonely Tuesday morning, ready to show me around a church I had travelled half the world to see. Thank you to Bob Taylor and Brian Woodlands for their help and advice in navigating Mr Floyd's prescriptions. I like to think that had Mr Floyd realised my book would include his work in 140 years' time, he might have been clearer in his penmanship and recipes.

A special acknowledgment must go to those I spend almost each day with – teachers and students alike, who are too polite to change the subject when it – *naturally* – turns to the insane. I cannot thank the English and History departments at my school enough for their support. A special nod to my Year 10 History class who allowed an entire lesson to be conducted solely about our favourite would-be assassin, George Morton. And to all of my other students who have not objected to the occasional (and yet highly relevant) tangent in class.

Thank you, also, to my family – particularly my parents, along with T, S, BE and ATC.

And finally, to the original patients and staff of Callan Park. Gifts of literature were often contributed to the hospital by well-wishers – and this book I donate to them with all my heart. Mental health has not quite lost its stigma yet, but I hope that in paying patients the attention soldiers, politicians, and other historical figures routinely receive, that I can give them the same sense of historical-justice. Many of the first patients at Callan Park went unmourned at their deaths, their families and friends living often overseas. I have visited the lonely sites of many of their graves – perhaps making me the first person to do so. This is their monument.

PREFACE

Ironmonger John Keep was outraged. A well-known and respected resident of Balmain in Sydney for more than a decade, in 1876 he discovered that the New South Wales government planned to build a lunatic asylum next door to him. John Keep's magnificent home was Broughton House, a beautiful two-storey manor house surrounded by wide open spaces, orchards, and other equally beautiful residences. The nearest was the mansion called Garryowen House, a few hundred metres up the hill towards Balmain Road. It was this house, in the middle of what had been recently re-named 'Callan Park', that Colonial Secretary Henry Parkes had decided would house lunatics.

In March 1876 a petition[1] against the asylum was put to the government by nine alarmed 'landowners in the vicinity of Garryowen'. Their arguments against the proposal were blunt. They said that they had all spent large amounts of money to buy into the quiet Balmain neighbourhood and furthermore to 'improve' their posh residences. This, they stressed, was reason enough not to subject them to the 'wild and dangerous antics of the insane' who, naturally, were assumed to be of a low, criminal class. The Balmain residents were perturbed that already some of the windows of Garryowen had been barred and that a wooden boundary wall had been erected at a height of seven feet. This, they declared, was surely not high enough to prevent the inevitable escape of the institution's inmates. With these amateur provisions, the nine accused the government of 'playing at mad-houses' and that such poor planning and decision-making would impact their lives – most notably the ladies' and children's – by the 'continual dread of violence and outrage' which must necessarily accompany such a design. As a last attempt to sway their perpetually-deaf audience the residents reminded the government of the 'sterile' nature of the soil at Callan Park, which was to ignore the heavy bounty of trees and orchards already there. They offered a snobbish solution: perhaps a location further 'inland' might be better chosen – or, that failing, that the lunatics might be housed at Dr Tucker's private asylum at Cook's River, for a mere £1 2s 6d per week, far *far* away from the pleasure grounds which were Callan Park. But their many concerns went unheeded. They lodged another petition at the end of March,[2] this time whipping up a frenzy with ninety-four signatures.[3] The New South Wales government ignored it again, as governments do, and a bare few months later Garryowen at Callan Park was established as a mad-house.

This situation was not a new one: in January 1859 the Victorian government had had a similar petition[4] brought against the use of the 'village reserve' at Kew in Melbourne as an asylum for the insane. A similar process had occurred too: the residents pointed out that they had spent a lot of money buying into their neighbourhood which they would never recoup if an asylum were built. The debate in the Victorian parliament even went so far as to discuss a site further away from the centre of Melbourne, made possible by railway lines. Politicians listened, and politicians ignored the residents' pleas. Kew Asylum was built.

It is easy, even for us safety ensconced in the twenty-first century, to sympathize with these alarmed neighbours of both Kew and Callan Park. Mad-houses, asylums, hospitals for the insane – we all know what these were like, thanks mainly to the vivid accounts which were common fodder to the sensational literature of the Victorian era: the same stories read by the residents of Kew and Balmain. Such novels are bursting at the seams with 'inconvenient' mothers, wives, fathers and husbands, carted off to some shady mad-house and shut away without hope or legal representation. Such was the focus of Charles Reade's 1863 novel *Hard Cash,* whose hero is incarcerated in a series of private asylums of varying quality – but all suffering the same defect: that they are slums of confinement and corruption, disease and greed, rather than therapy and cure. Importantly, and frighteningly, none of the 'doctors' can see – or wish to acknowledge – that Reade's hero is in fact sane, but being framed by his Machiavellian father and uncle. Thus un-blinkered by any mental illness, Reade's hero is intensely aware of the malpractice and sadistic treatment used to contain inmates including himself. Given festering food, regularly beaten, confined with heavy bolted doors and never allowed outside, the treatment of Reade's hero was designed by the author to enlighten the reading public of the conditions faced by patients in England's asylums. Along with other novels of the time, it created a blinding image of all insane institutions as realms of sadistic brutality, where humanity was easily forgotten in the quest for a profit.

But it was not only the doctors and their gaol-like institutions which were to be mistrusted. Most often depicted as irrationally violent, rather than merely depressed as was the much more common reality, all patients – even women – were to be feared, as in the secret attic-dwelling Bertha Mason in *Jane Eyre*:

> *The maniac bellowed: she parted her shaggy locks from her visage, and gazed wildly at her visitors. I recognised well that purple face, – those bloated features. Mrs. Poole advanced.*
> *'Keep out of the way,' said Mr. Rochester, thrusting her aside: 'she has no knife now, I suppose, and I'm on my guard.'*
> *'One never knows what she has, sir: she is so cunning: it is not in mortal discretion to fathom her craft.'*

The reality – the horror – of Victorian health care for the mentally unwell is clearly conveyed in these texts. Of course, not every madman encountered such abuse – there were good asylums too, headed by sympathetic doctors with caring staff. But it is the darker side which we are much more interested in. The evidence of mistreatment in such nineteenth century institutions is well-known and has gone down in popular history. Weekend trips to Bedlam in London, where a tourist could pay a small entrance fee to ogle at the patients caged within, speak volumes about the popular attitude towards the mad. John Perceval's famous account of his own incarceration in various English asylums, where he managed to essentially cure his own schizophrenia, despite harsh treatment, is another:

Though in a highly nervous and excitable state, I was subjected to witness the insults and cruel outrages practised on other lunatics by the keepers, and from one to another. I have seen two old men thrown on the floor, one of sixty-nine years of age struck a violent blow on the kidneys; he had a complaint there; one insulted and ridiculed by the servants. I saw one young lunatic strangled before my eyes till the face was swollen with blood, and his eyes started out of their sockets; I used to see this same young gentleman daily confined to a small court for exercise, often fastened to a seat out of doors; I know he was not supplied with paper for the privy ...

Perceval published his account of his both mistreatment and successes in 1840, entitled *A Narrative of the Treatment Experienced by a Gentleman During a State of Mental Derangement.* Like Reade, he hoped to shed light onto the treatment of men and women in England's mad-houses.

But these fictional and real accounts, sometimes designed to initiate at least a public outcry, and at most governmental change, have blackened all nineteenth century asylums and their doctors. History has not been kind to psychiatric care: historians are all too quick to shrug and judge all mad-houses as necessarily fiscally-motivated, all doctors and attendants malevolent and sexual predators who found joy and power in perpetuating the misery of the mentally unwell. But was this horrific treatment of the mentally unwell actually the case at Callan Park?

Journalists in particular find time a difficult concept to grasp: one only has to google 'Callan Park' to find that the reputation of nineteenth century institutions – both specifically Callan Park and more broadly speaking – has been tainted by mid twentieth century versions.

In 1961 the Honourable Mr Justice McClemens completed his enquiry into various matters concerning Callan Park. The Royal Commission which he headed had been designed to look into the conditions endured by both patients and employees, but focused primarily on the 'allegations of brutality, theft, drunkenness and neglect of duty by the Callan Park Mental Hospital staff'.[5] The Royal Commission had been long awaited: calls for such an investigation had grown more vigorous two decades previously in the 1940s, with claims that patients were out of control, being offered only limited medical help for their conditions due to the significant overcrowding of the institution, being sexually assaulted, forced to work long hours into the night and were regularly assaulted by kicks to the head.[6] It was only in 1960 when Callan Park's new medical superintendent, Dr Bailey, became whistle-blower, that a Commission was initiated. After a hearing spanning seven months, Justice McClemens found Callan Park staff seriously wanting in professionalism. In his official report, he found that there was substantial evidence of thieving by staff from both medicinal and food stores, deep corruption and a culture of laziness and carelessness among nurses, attendants and medical officers. Further, that the hospital was under-staffed, particularly in terms of medical practitioners. McClemens' report urged a drastic reduction in patient numbers, renovations be conducted throughout the dilapidated buildings, and better training for staff. This, he said, would allow for 'active treatment or rehabilitation' rather than the stagnating 'care' and bullying which existed at the time.[7]

Calls in the 1940s, 50s and 60s for a Royal Commission have been somehow mis-imagined to have been simmering from Callan Park's inception in the 1870s. Headlines from today make that clear: 'Victorian psychiatric patients' grim fate in hellish 1800s hospitals' and 'Sydney's shameful asylums: The silent houses of pain where inmates were chained and sadists reigned'.[8] This book's aim is not to call into question the wrongs committed by staff – and patients – in Callan Park's twentieth century existence. It is to question whether Callan Park's *beginnings* were honourable and, importantly, helpful to the hundreds of patients who walked its corridors, slept in its dormitories and found contentment in its farm and cricket pitch – or not.

NOTE ON THE SOURCES

The bulk of the research for this book has been from the primary sources associated with Callan Park. The Lunacy Acts required accurate records to be kept of the happenings in all of the asylums in New South Wales. This bureaucracy consisted of many books and journals which were frequently updated to record the events at the hospital by the various managers. Many of these files, however, have been lost or culled at some point before they reached their secure home at the State Records Authority of New South Wales. Even those which now are cared for at the Records Authority have been badly damaged by carelessness or water at some point or other, and occasionally important information has been obscured. There is something very transporting about reading these files however: holding the heavy tomes frequently referred to by each of the medical superintendents – Manning, Scholes, Blaxland, Ross – and straining to read their archaic handwriting is a very special experience indeed.

Callan Park's *Medical Case Books* are happily all intact for the timeframe of this book, though damaged in some parts. The *Medical Case Books* are large leather-bound volumes frequently with peeling spines and faded gold capitalised labels. They have marbled endpapers and the sheets within have an aged brownish colouring these days. Patients were given a double-page spread and were ordered according to date of admission. When these two pages were filled a new double-page spread was found in the next available book, with a note at the end of the first pages directing the reader to the next book which housed the continuation. As a result, patients who were resident at Callan Park for several decades had their notes spread over numerous volumes. Patients who were discharged and readmitted also had their histories volumes-apart, but with no note at the end of a discharge leading the reader to his next admission pages. For a time the doctors at Callan Park changed this system and provided patients with four pages in a volume in the hope that more than this would not be needed, and the patients' notes would be thus contained. This appears to have been stopped due to the waste of paper occurring as a result. In the 1900s a more economical system was adopted and patients were allocated brown folders and all relevant notes were thus collected.

These books are magnificent artefacts of New South Wales' early medical history. On the left hand page of each double-page spread was recorded the patient's full name (including any aliases), age, social condition, number of children, occupation, nativity, residence, religion, form of mental disorder, supposed cause of the disorder, duration of the attack, details of any previous attack, date of last admission (if any), details of insane relations, and the date of discharge (which could mean cure, transfer to another hospital, or death). Under this compact and brief moment of biographical details, the rest of the page consists of blank lines where details of 'Mental and Bodily Condition, Symptoms &c.' were recorded. The doctors were obliged to offer a description of the patient as their first observation, in the case that a description was ever needed to locate an escapee or judge an identity. In the late 1800s other information concerning pulse, height, weight and bowel-regularity was also included. After this followed the observations carried out while the patient existed in the Admissions Ward. Successive entries were filled out regularly but not terribly frequently – often once every three months unless a particularly noteworthy incident occurred. This was in accordance with the 1878 Lunacy Act which ordered that,

> *During the first month after admission, entries to be made at least once in every week, and oftener when the nature of the case requires it. Afterwards, in recent or acute cases, entries to be made at least in every month; and in chronic cases, subject to little variation, at least once in every three months.*

At Callan Park this was carried out fully, though quite often the comment 'no change' was the only record entered for multiple months in a row. On the right-hand page of the spread was space for information regarding the date the patient was admitted to Callan Park, the folio number (one folio consisted of two pages) and the 'No. On Register' which was sometimes used to track some patients through the files. 'Further History' was also furnished at the top of this page, and often copied the ticket which accompanied patients from Reception House, the transient asylum where most patients were initially held pending their admission to one of the hospitals for the insane. Treatments, including prescriptions, and information as to diet and allowances, were also recorded here.

While the information contained in these volumes has furnished a large part of this book, many of the details – namely their marital status, number of children, occupation etc – have required confirmation. One patient, Rev Frederick Legard, was allocated a wife he certainly never had during his life; another, Fillipo Parcelli, had no wife on paper, where he certainly did have one in reality – and a child too. It is unclear whether the Callan Park staff were making clerical errors, guessing as to the answers – a Church of England reverend would be likely to have had a wife, for instance – or that patients were providing information that was wrong (either due to confusion or resentment at being confined). Garton cites numerous examples of men and women calling themselves 'Loony' or 'Turd' and this being entered into the state's records as accurate despite its obvious error.[1] The same issues plague the records of Reception House, whose staff were frequently forced to amend the names of patients – perhaps after the initial violence of being admitted. The process seems to have been a verbal one – Legard was called 'Lingard' initially, and the two names, particularly when spoken by a disturbed mind doubled with a thick Yorkshire accent, might sound similar. It is unclear who recorded the information in these books. References *to* the medical superintendent rule out the head of the asylum. It is likely the attendant in charge of the ward had input, along with the dispenser who filled in the right-hand side pages.

The four groups of twelve which formed the first swell of Garryowen in 1879 were transferred with a special set of handwritten summaries from Gladesville Asylum, and which still survive in the bottom of a dirty box at the State Records Authority of New South Wales. No other transfers seem to have been furnished with these, and it is possible that these large groups were unusual in this respect. There are four bundles, each secured by a rusting metal split pin. The bundles contain a sheet detailing the patient 'Before Admission', 'On Admission' to Gladesville and 'Present Condition'. These notes were directly transcribed into the Callan Park *Medical Case Books.* Many of the patients' blue Lunacy Warrants, documents not terribly useful in illuminating the patient's exact condition, were also attached to these, though those who had been at Gladesville for more than a few months had had their warrants pasted into a magnificent scrap book the size of a small refrigerator. A table of each patient's property was also included but this was not recorded anywhere in Callan Park's books.

The hospital's *Medical Journals* are also a rich source of information. Large and relatively thin books, these also were leather bound with beautiful papers. They were written in by the medical superintendent and were a summary of the major incidents in the hospital each week. Callan Park's do not begin until September 1879 when the first group of twelve men was transferred from Gladesville to join the original forty-four at Garryowen. These double-pages were ruled up in a table: on the left were columns to record the total number of patients at Callan Park, along with the statistics and names of those under restraint (which included camisoles or muffs) and those in seclusion, along with details of their misbehaviour. On the right page were columns detailing the number of patients under medical treatment (sorted into Male and Female columns), and finally Details of Deaths, Injuries and Violence to Patients Since Last Entry, and General Observations (which included banal details about the weather affecting epileptics, along with the names of patients discharged and newly admitted).

Much of Callan Park's correspondence – letters both about, and from, patients – has been culled and those records which remain are random specimens. Apart from anything else, letters written by delusional patients were often not sent and the Inspector General of the Insane, Frederic Norton Manning in his annual *Reports* recounted his perusal of these, noting their destruction in accordance with the Lunacy Act. It is interesting to note –

particularly in the case of George Morton, who attempted the assassination of Queen Victoria in 1872 and who was possibly incarcerated in the stone 'cell' in Garryowen's basement – that some of these were actually kept and still exist today. Thus the correspondence which survives is a random motley assortment and is often so full of untruths that is was decided by staff unwise to send to relatives. Its use in illuminating the reality of nineteenth century Callan Park is therefore compromised.

In surveying the records which survive from other hospitals contemporary with Callan Park, it is clear that many items from Callan Park have been lost or destroyed. Callan Park's *Post Mortem Registers* are no more, the Patients' *Leave of Absence Registers* are gone; records of printing, and – most disappointingly – the records of the addresses of patients' friends, are also missing.

Gaol records from the time have also been used in this history and illuminate well the condition of some of the patients inclined to violence and mischievousness. New South Wales' gaols at this time were just beginning to enhance their inmate records through the photographing of criminals. The wholesale lack of photographs of even the most violent criminal inmates of Callan Park suggest a ban on photographing lunatics at the time. Even those charged with some misdemeanour were not pictorially recorded. Images of patients are therefore difficult to find and rely on them being named in group portraits. Few, even, were of a class high enough for painted portraits to be a viable avenue of research.

PART ONE
THE HOSPITAL

1

CALLAN PARK: BRANCH ESTABLISHMENT AND THE 'FIRST FORTY-FOUR'

Ignoring the protests of John Keep and his neighbours, Garryowen House at Callan Park was made a branch establishment of Gladesville Hospital for the Insane in 1876, just as Yarra Bend had been in 1848. This was a significant moment for Dr Frederic Norton Manning and his Lunacy Department, as it was the first step to establishing Callan Park as New South Wales' – and Australia's – premier hospital for the mentally ill.

The first residents were forty-four men, chosen especially upon the basis of their temperament and skills. It was the facilities which dictated the choice of these patients: firstly, due to the limited security of the site, and perhaps the fears only recently voiced by the ninety-four neighbours in their petition, these men were necessarily of a low maintenance category of care. They were either of advanced age or calm disposition – or both – and were, as such, 'safe' choices as the first Callan Park residents: unlikely to be loud, disruptive or to attempt escape. In this way, one might say they were a PR-dream. The two primary types of insanity in this group were dementia and mania, with smaller numbers diagnosed with melancholia, imbecility and one as suffering from 'general insanity'. The second reason for the choice of these men were that their skills were to be put to use in readying the house for a future increase in numbers, but also in the quest to make the place homely for themselves. Hence, tradesmen and painters were some of the first chosen to occupy the new hospital; others, who could write, were put to good use in the office. In the group of primarily labourers, there was also a porter, a shoemaker, a wheelwright, a tutor, several storekeepers and miners, a farmer, a clergyman, a publisher, a tailor, a publican and a bank clerk. Of the forty-four, twenty-eight were aged over forty, with nine of these in excess of sixty-one years of age. The majority were recorded as single, and only eighteen married. Twenty-four were Church of England, eighteen Roman Catholic and one pagan (with one unlisted). Approximately one third each were from New South Wales, England and Ireland. The rest hailed from Wales, China and Scotland.

One of the new hospital's most interesting original patients was the aged Frederick Legard.[1] A gentleman, having studied mathematics and classics at Cambridge, Legard stood at a height of five feet eight inches. He had dark, intelligent eyes, and distinguished greying hair which framed his sharp, inherited features. Before being committed to Callan Park as a pauper madman, he had been a well-connected vicar ministering his Baronet family's seat in the far north of Yorkshire in England.

Like his fellow transferees, the lunatic Legard was chosen for Garryowen based on his behaviour: he was quiet and well-conducted in his daily routine, but he could also read and write – something which the small staff at Callan Park found quite useful. In his Gladesville *Medical Case Book*, Legard was described as making himself 'very useful in the office' at the branch establishment at Garryowen, and when the first forty-four were 'officially' made Callan Park's first patients in 1878, when Callan Park split from Gladesville and became an institution in and of itself, it is highly likely that it was Legard, who left his own name until last, who wrote up each patient's medical details in the new *Medical Case Books*. He was described as being 'very quiet and well-conducted but is an odd peculiar man'. Callan Park and Legard agreed with each other: he was safe, cared for and well-fed. As a result, his eccentricities became his foremost symptoms, and the violence he had exhibited in the past, evaporated. It was noticed that he was 'addicted to physicking himself for imaginary ailments'. This was summarised by the staff at Callan Park, who wrote: 'he gradually calmed down [after a time at Gladesville] and for a long time the chief symptoms have been those of eccentricity'. At sixty-five, he was one of the elders of the new hospital. He had status among the patients as one who could not only read and write, but one who was allowed to assist in the office. He also helped in the store where provisions and other items such as utensils – a valuable commodity for any patient intent on escape or suicide – were held. For this he received extra allowances in butter and brandy – a luxury for a man with not a penny to his name.

Legard as one of the 'first forty-four' found Garryowen House much as it had been during the time of its earlier private owners, Brenan and Gordon, and many of its fine features still exist today. It is a tall, two-storey sandstone mansion with a verandah along the front side of the house, shaded by large virulent trees. The sloping roof of this neatly-tiled space leads the eye upwards to the first floor, pierced with many windows – which at the time would have been barred. Certainly, small alterations had been made to the place to make it work as a hospital, but most of it went unchanged in the first year or so.

The choice of calm patients seems to have been well-anticipated. In the medical records of these patients, including Legard, there are remarkably brief entries which give no indication of any issues arising at Garryowen. Comments such as 'has been at the Callan Park branch establishment for some months now' abound in these men's records. With the lack of reports from newspapers of disturbances at Callan Park, or escaped lunatics terrifying the local residents, we are left to believe that the first couple of years were unremarkable. So too the medical progress of these patients: the staff were much too busy painting the house and tending to the gardens to take time to update the medical files.

In September 1877, after these forty-four had been in residence for a little over a year, the government called for tenders[2] for the temporary buildings which were to be constructed as extensions to the rear of Garryowen. To John Keep and his neighbours, this would have been a sign of the government's and Manning's satisfaction with the state of affairs at Callan Park and their willingness to expand there. The plans included the extension of the front verandah 'to make a pleasant promenade for its inmates',[3] and the addition of extra wards on the south side. Out-buildings including a stable and laundry were also to be built,[4] though none survive today.

At this point Callan Park was still a branch establishment of Gladesville Hospital and not yet an institution in its own right. It depended upon Gladesville for its staffing and administration, and was managed by the Head of the Lunacy Department and soon to be Inspector General of the Insane, Dr Frederic Norton Manning, Gladesville's medical superintendent at the time. There were no medical officers directly attached to Callan Park yet, but rather visiting medical men from Gladesville made frequent tours of the branch establishment and didn't update the patient files. The staff which was at Callan Park was a small one.

In 1876 there was an officer in charge, most likely an experienced attendant chosen by Manning, who was allowed accommodation and provisions besides his salary of £100 per annum. His salary was increased to £120 in October 1877. This is very likely to have been William Henry Little who in the 1878 *Government Gazette* was listed as chief attendant and receiving the same salary. Little lived at Callan Park with his wife and children for several decades before retiring in the early twentieth century. A man of medium height and sporting a thick Victorian moustache, in 1915 he received the Imperial Service Medal for his loyalty to the civil service. Under him were two senior attendants, one arriving in April and the other in May of 1876, who earned £78 per year – raised to £90 the following year – on top of their accommodation and provisions; and two residential junior attendants at £72 per annum – and increased to three the following year. Besides these indoor attendants, there was a Gardner, Samuel Cheetham, who lived on site and who was paid £66 per year. The female cook and the laundress also lived at Garryowen and were paid £50 and £46 respectively. These women are likely to have also been engaged as cleaners to undertake general domestic duties. They would have been in constant contact with the patients, some of whom would have assisted in food preparation, and the washing and drying of the immense amount of laundry such a place would create. Two Chaplains appointed by the Colonial Secretary, one Church of England and one Roman Catholic, both paid £26 per year, rounded out the staff. In the first few years, these were Rev W. F. B. Uzzell and Rev John Forrest. At this point in Callan Park's history, no nurses – male or female – were employed. Medical care was conducted by the superintendent and visiting medical officers and any ongoing care would have been administered by the attendants.

In August 1878 Callan Park was officially cut from Gladesville and became an asylum in its own right. The first forty-four were officially discharged from Gladesville and admitted to Callan Park, though they had been resident for two years. The original letter[5] formally acknowledging this is still in existence and serves as an interesting piece of pre-Federation bureaucracy:

> *To Frederic Norton Manning, Esquire M.D. the Medical Superintendent of the Lunatic Asylum at Tarban Creek and to Frederic Norton Manning Esquire MD the Medical Superintendent of the Lunatic Asylum at Callan Park.*
>
> *Whereas by the Lunacy Act, 1869, the Colonial Secretary is empowered by writing under his had, to order and direct the removal of any Lunatic other than a Criminal Lunatic, from any Asylum or Licensed House to any other Asylum or Licensed House; and whereas* [names of the first forty-four] *are Lunatics other than Criminal Lunatics, and are now detained in the Lunatic Asylum at Tarban Creek and it is desirable that the said forty four lunatics should be removed thence to the Lunatic Asylum at Callan Park.*
>
> *Now I Michael Fitzpatrick the Colonial Secretary by virtue of the power given to me by the said Act, do, by this writing, order and direct the removal of the said forty four lunatics from the said Lunatic Asylum at Tarban Creek to the said Lunatic Asylum at Callan Park.*
>
> *Given under my hand in duplicate, at the Colonial Secretary's Office Sydney this twenty fifth day of July 1878.*

At the beginning of August, less than a week later, Callan Park's administration started up in earnest. This must have been a hectic time:

Callan Park was no longer playing second fiddle to Gladesville – now, records needed to be kept, patients' files updated, provisions ordered. The place would have been in a state of chaos with builders erecting the extra weatherboard wards on the site. For some time this continued, until September 1879, when the first incarnation of Callan Park was complete and was 'by no means unpicturesque'.[6]

Entering the front door of Garryowen via the shaded verandah, a visitor would arrive in a spacious and grand hall or refectory, cool even on a hot Sydney afternoon. On the western side, or to the visitor's right, was the old drawing room, now the 'Edith Wright Room' of the Writers' Centre and for the patients, a library and visitors' room. This room was papered in the same pattern which still exists in small amounts under glass in the Edith Wright Room – a beige and white floral pattern – of the 'pulp' wallpaper type. 'Pulp' is thus referred to because of its relative cheapness to produce. The pattern is printed directly onto the paper without any background colour. It is also of a type which is less prone to water damage, and hence easily cleaned.[7] The room would have been lined with shelves full of the books and periodicals regularly donated by well-wishers including the Free Public Library, unclaimed newspapers from General Post Office[8] and illustrated books from locals.[9] There is some evidence to suggest that it was not only novels which lined the shelves – mathematical and academic works were supplied to quench Legard's thirst. In accordance with Manning's philosophy, trinkets and ornaments would have been displayed on the walls and tables, creating a thoroughly home-like effect. The floor was covered in cocoa-nut matting and, in the middle of the room, there was a billiard table which could be flipped to make an ordinary table.[10]

The remainder of the ground floor of Garryowen, besides the offices, kitchen and pantry, made up Ward One. The numbering system which Callan Park adopted was in line with Gladesville's system and indicated the temperament of the patient thus within. One was generally for convalescent patients, Two for violent and noisy patients. Opposite the library, on the left-hand side of the hall, was a dormitory of twenty beds where Legard would have initially slept. These, too, would have been cosy and comfortable, particularly as it was the weatherboard extensions which were to house the violent and epileptic patients, and in this ward opposite the library, a much quieter and convalescent type of patient found sanctuary.

Ward One further accommodated a dining room which sat fifty patients and was entered by a French window from the airing court or garden at the back of the house, near the spring. All meals would have been taken here and, given the type of patient treated in this area, meals would have been on the whole uninterrupted and quite civilised. Leading out of this dining parlour was a day room, 'a large, light, airy apartment furnished with everything that [would] conduce to the comfort of the inmates'.[11] Here were more London and Colonial magazines and books, along with games and other amusements.

The magnificent floating stone staircase which is currently the means to access the upper floors of the New South Wales Writers' Centre is the same one which existed in 1879 as a way to the first floor of the Callan Park Asylum.[12] This second storey housed a bathroom, along with more patient wards, this time for further well-behaved and trusted patients, who were allowed to keep a small box containing their best suit and knick-knacks.[13] The fact that these patients were allowed to keep clothes – particularly trousers – and not have these confiscated at night, recommended them as patients who had never tried to escape, or shown any willingness to assist others in such an endeavour. The lack of pants was often all that stood between a patient eager to escape out a window in the middle of the night and liberation. It is also possible that these men were from the 'better classes'. These patients, in 1882, received carpets on the floors, and mosquito curtains.[14] Their rooms were painted half with blue and half with brown and 'prettily stencilled with various colours in a tasteful design' by the patients themselves.[15] It is likely that these patients paid for this privilege.

Near these patients' rooms was the accommodation of the attendants. The limited evidence connected to the attendants' quarters suggests that rooms were small but comfortable. An image from 1903,[16] not in Garryowen House but elsewhere in the later hospital, known as the Kirkbride Complex, shows a neatly made bed surrounded by numerous ornaments including photo frames. In 1881, at Garryowen, there was a fire in one attendant's room caused by the gas pendant on the ceiling becoming either unscrewed or broken and setting fire to the wooden roof;[17] this room was undoubtedly one of the apartments on the first floor. Fire was a constant worry in any asylum, but through this incident it was realised that Callan Park's height meant that the site's low water pressure would be useless in the event of a large fire.[18] The solution was to keep buckets filled with water and long-handled mops in each ward, each night,[19] since even the water supply could not be completely guaranteed, with the City Engineer being called on several occasions to reconnect the supply.[20]

In this quiet atmosphere of Garryowen and Ward One were also the offices of Callan Park's second medical superintendent. This was the vastly humane Dr Richard Battersby Scholes. Scholes and his clerk, along with the chief attendant Little, all had their offices on this floor. A journalist who visited Callan Park in 1880 described Scholes' clerk in great detail, though he does not appear to have been registered as one of Callan Park's patients:

> *The fittings of this room are extremely elaborate. It contains two writing bureaux, one of which is the Doctor's, and the other that of his clerk – a patient, who, I am happy to chronicle, has recovered under Dr Scholes's intelligent treatment. This man is an extraordinary genius in the way of manufacturing odds and ends, and many samples of is work embellish the office. This poor fellow, besides having suffered mental aberration is likewise afflicted with deafness. Dr Scholes, however, having heard of the new invention, the audiophone, has contrived to manufacture one, and the simple little machine has proved a great success. The patient, it would appear, was formerly mate of a ship, but left his vessel, for some reason, and resolved to pursue his fortunes on shore. He was not, however, successful in obtaining employment, and the many disappointments he experienced brought on melancholia. Subsequently, feeling an irresistible longing to destroy himself coming over him, he surrendered himself to the authorities for protection. In appearance the man in decidedly prepossessing – his*

bearing being frank, open, and manly. It is to be hoped that when he is discharged by [Head of the Lunacy Department, Inspector General of the Insane] *Dr Manning (which, I am told, will be very shortly) some benevolent person will take him by the hand, and by giving him a lift on the highway of life, prevent a recurrence of the poor fellow's misfortune.*[21]

Scholes was Callan Park's second medical superintendent after Manning, and ran the new institution from 1879 to 1881, receiving an annual salary of £450. He was well-trained in the ways of the state's asylums, having also worked at Gladesville and Parramatta. In 1881 when he resigned, he went to Queensland to head the asylum at Goodna and the Lunacy Department of Queensland.[22] The job, while prestigious, was not an envied one. A writer for the *Sydney Morning Herald* described the situation thus:[23]

Dr. Patrick Smith, superintendent of the Woogaroo Lunatic Asylum, has resigned. He is an excellent doctor I believe, though not so good a business manager. The immediate cause of his resignation was some difference he had with his medical subordinate; but I fancy that the bitter and persistent attacks made on him by some Ms. L. A. had a great deal to do with it. His successor will be Dr. R. B. Scholes, from the Callan Park Asylum in your colony. If he does not quarrel with influential Ipswitch politicians he will do well.

By his death in 1898, which was unexpected, Scholes was regarded as a high authority on insanity and personally popular.[24] Scholes' reign over Callan Park was a calm one. The files from his time were well managed, and there was a particular lack of restraint used while he was medical superintendent.

Leaving the relative peace and safety of Garryowen was Ward Two, housed in the temporary weatherboard buildings attached to the south of the mansion. This ward was for the refractory and epileptic patients and included twenty single rooms along with a number of associated dormitories. Single rooms were the preferred method of housing such violent patients as they allowed for segregation when required, and also allowed for the seclusion of some by the closing of the door to their room. For patients prone to escape, single rooms were provided as a means of limiting their ability to make accomplices of others. In 1882 several of the window panes in Ward Two were replaced with wire netting to reduce the number of injuries sustained by violent patients breaking the glass. In 1883, after the success of this, more were converted, with the note that no rain entered the rooms since they all faced north.[25]

Such a system seems at odds with Reade and Perceval's thoughts on asylums as places of brutality and discomfort. To be sure, Callan Park was a state institution unhampered by the distracting need to make a profit, as the boutique private enterprises which star in their books required. But if one departs for a moment from the happy and content world of *above* stairs, and moves *downstairs* to the basement of Garryowen, an entirely different picture is formed of treatment under Manning's watch. Basements in houses of this era are not unusual – but the use of a basement for the seclusion of patients is notable. Garryowen's basement is quite curious in its own right. Spanning the entire space under what was originally the library and dining room, the place is large and not altogether unhomely. Constructed of solid stone and of a height which would permit most men to stand, the place is well-ventilated by metal gratings along the western side. There is even a small fireplace there. One patient – whose preference for falsehoods is important to keep in mind – in 1883 complained[26] of being kept in a 'stone cell' while at Garryowen during a time when he was considered dangerous and unpredictable: 'I sleep very well. – I am in a cell ... This portends very bad. I was put in it by [the medical superintendent]. I was troubled by religion – and voices'. This particular patient, George Morton, was at the time being famously kept exclusively in the weatherboard Ward Two. Importantly, the rooms here were made of wood, with the exception of the single rooms, which were made of brick.[27] The patient, whose insanity had climaxed in a strange attempt at taking Queen Victoria's life in London in 1872, wrote further that,

The shadow of death is on me; and I am treated as a felon. They cannot deny it. What do they mean by placing me in a cell? To drive me mad with terror? – Every artifice which villainy and fraud could think of, has been tried upon me, by the Government, to drive me raving mad, for ever, but they don't succeed. No There are ten thousand pounds, worse patients, here, than me; and they are permitted to sleep in large rooms, with beds, although perfect Demoniacs, and not safe one from another. While I a perfect convalescent from syphallus have to lay in a stone cell by myself and no one within call; If I was to knock till death was on me ...

It is easy, and tempting, to jump at this and call into question all of Manning's work. Was he responsible for this part of his 'hospital'? If the basement at Garryowen *was* used to contain patients, our questions should tend towards those concerning the use of the space, and for what reasons it might have been utilized. Was Morton being *punished* by being housed in the 'cell'? Was he allowed light and fresh air, as exists today in this area of the house? How long was he in seclusion? Under whose authority could he be admitted – and could this have been subject to corruption? Or was such a space – quiet and calm – the ideal place in which to subdue a maniacal outburst? During my own visit to the basement, on a day when the house was full of perhaps two dozen people, their voices and movements were clearly audible – and I did not doubt that my own voice could be heard by them, above. Was Morton actually not so far from help, and was perhaps being monitored without his knowledge? The access to the basement sits under the floating staircase in the main hall and it is difficult to see how shouts – screams – could not be heard by patients, visitors and staff below. Much more likely is that Morton was housed in a brick single room – at ground or first floor level.

In late 1879 Callan Park's two-ward system was ready for its first increase in patients. The first forty-four, chosen for their docility and skills in painting, crafting and gardening, had created a utopia of state-run psychiatric treatment. Now the hospital began accepting new patients from the over-crowded Gladesville, along with single admissions from other sources. The Gladesville transfers were done slowly, in four groups of twelve from between September and December. It is unclear why these groups were transferred in dozens – but perhaps it has something to do with their mode of travel. There are no clear indications from the sources of the time which are specific in explaining how patients arrived at Callan Park. Callan Park's extensive stables might indicate carts as the fetcher of admissions. Indeed, the early patients seemed acutely aware of the way back to Gladesville by foot, which indicates that transfers were possibly made by road. Half an hour after his transfer from Gladesville to Callan Park in 1879, patient Charles Wilkie escaped by merely retracing the route he had just taken to arrive.[28] Callan Parks' proximity to water – in connection with Parramatta, Gladesville and the Reception House at Darlinghurst – also suggests another possible option. Indeed, Gladesville's early patients arrived by the 'Bedlam Ferry'.[29] In 1875 there was some considerable irritation on the part of both Manning and the public at the use of public steamers on the Parramatta River being used to shift patients between Gladesville and Parramatta Asylums.[30] It is, however, difficult to envisage the more violent and refractory patients making travel a simple matter, and at Callan Park the substantial walk up the hill, from the water to Garryowen, would not have been an easy one for the attendants.

The four groups of twelve arrived from Gladesville were not of the same nature to the first forty-four, and there was a substantial time needed by all to accommodate these newcomers. Some of the original patients, hereto well-behaved, found the arrival of the new patients too much, and several relapsed. During the three months of new arrivals, Henry Black, a convalescent, wandered away for the first time in his significant period of care and was found in Pyrmont. William Brennan, a new arrival and sufferer of vivid religious delusions, began his career as a master escapee with attendants and police forced to focus days of surveillance on his brother's house, wherein he was secreted. In December Frederick Legard, the elderly clergyman, joined in with three violent newcomers in a co-ordinated and premeditated attack on his ward attendants.[31]

Besides their temperament, these 'forty-eight' patients were of a similar mix to the original forty-four: they were labourers, sawyers, butchers, gardeners, masons, blacksmiths and even a medical student. Overall, however, they were a little younger, with nineteen aged between twenty-one and thirty. The majority were again from England, Ireland and New South Wales, but this time many more nationalities were also included: more Chinese, an American, a German, an Italian and a Frenchman, two Scots and one from 'unknown' origin. Again, most patients were either demented, melancholic or maniacal – but these maniacs were particularly violent and aggressive and needed especial care to avoid their escape. This was an issue with Callan Park from the beginning: the seven foot fence which had so alarmed John Keep as easily scalable turned out indeed to be so, and many escapees used this to its full extent.[32] Into the mix of these new arrivals were thrown two patients suffering from the 'general paralysis of the insane' (known more commonly as late-stage syphilis), a disease infamous for its paranoia and subsequent violence.

Like some of his fellows during this upheaval, Legard relapsed. The calm life Garryowen had previously supplied was shattered by the arrival of these four dozen new men, many of whom were violent and refractory patients. The quiet surroundings previously enjoyed by Legard, removed from noise and aggravation, and surrounded by fields very like what he had enjoyed in rural North Yorkshire as a boy, was interrupted. In November of 1879, after two dozen new patients had arrived, and a month before the other twenty-four came, Legard was removed from Ward One and transferred quickly to Ward Two. He had killed one of the hospital's pets. The majority of the asylum's animals were farm animals or birds, and in his notes there was no elaboration concerning species or method. Clearly, however, the event was severe enough to remove him to the weatherboard extensions beside Garryowen, to the ward which also came to house the dangerous African Khumis Baroot, Italian Fillipo Parcelli and the would-be assassin George Morton. It is tempting for the modern reader to suspect that this kind of event was not unusual – surely placing tame animals near such men was one temptation too far? But rare was the destruction of that element of Moral Therapy which the patients saw each day and which created for them a home rather than an asylum. In 1879 Manning addressed this directly, defending his choices of decoration and homeliness in his institutions: 'How seldom are the pictures, looking-glasses, and ornaments of different kinds broken or defaced. How rarely are the birds and animals in the wards wantonly injured; whilst interruption or disorder at the amusements of religious services is almost unknown'.[33]

As more patients arrived, Legard became worse. He directed his violence towards other inmates and was often secluded in a single room in order to calm him. As a member of a working party involved in painting the walls of the weatherboard side of the hospital, he suffered a sudden turn and was secluded for 'disfiguring the walls' which his fellow patients had worked hard to perfect. In a fight with another patient he earned himself a black eye, and in the surrounding days began to lose much weight. In December 1879 he was one of four, along with Fillipo Parcelli, William Clancy and Samuel Payne, who launched an attack on the attendants of Ward Two and even after seclusion for four and a half hours, was still violent the next day and was locked in his room again from 10am to 3pm. Three days later he renewed his attack with another patient, William Brennan, striking an attendant, and again he was secluded. At the beginning of 1880 he was in a fight with a patient named Robson and in February, being 'noisy and quarrelsome' he was secluded for another four hours. But if Ward Two initially exacerbated his troubled mind, it also came to soothe it: soon Legard was described as 'quieter' and 'much better', working well and sleeping consistently. He was still collecting 'all kinds of rubbish and [was] at times noisy and quarrelsome' but he was putting on weight again. Odd occasions of disturbance earned him time locked in his room – like when he was punished for 'disturbing the church services'. Perhaps however, on this occasion, we might forgive the ex-clergyman's opinion of the meagre services at early Callan Park.

In 1881 Legard sustained a serious injury to his ankle as a result of a struggle with one of the Ward Two attendants, James Veitch. Like both Parcelli and Baroot, Legard had developed an obsession with clothes – particularly those of other patients. Baroot was rather prone to stealing clothes, and

Parcelli had issues with wearing them – particularly hats and shoes. Legard was described in his notes as being 'in the habit of taking other patients' clothes and is usually violent if he is required to give them up'. Whether this particular characteristic was a learned behaviour from his homeless days in the Domain, a behaviour copied off other patients at Garryowen or merely an indication that Legard found Callan Park a cold place to be, is unclear. On the morning of the incident, in mid-May, Legard rose from bed and put on two pairs of trousers. Veitch taking issue with this, there was a struggle which ended in Legard's ankle being sprained. As a result of this pain, the patient spat in Veitch's face and struck him; when the two fell together, attendant Love arrived and assisted by restraining Legard by the arm. The attendant in charge of the ward, Sherack, informed the medical superintendent of the event. Throughout the inquiry, then begun by the medical superintendent, Veitch maintained that Legard, having previously taken another patient's pants, was being asked to give them up when he refused and attacked the attendant. Legard, on the other hand, accused Veitch of knocking him down before forcibly removing the trousers over his boots, and that the twisting associated with this had injured his ankle. Dr Scholes disagreed with Legard, concluding that the injury was more likely the result of the fall. No one was blamed.

In this early time, the odd patient was admitted outside these co-ordinated transfers. One of these was William Taylor,[34] a 10-year-old from Kingston who was admitted into the ranks of these sometimes intimidating and unpredictable men. Very few children were admitted to Callan Park, and it is quite unsettling to read in his records his answers to biographical questions meant for adults, such as occupation and social condition. In response to this issue in Victoria, Kew Asylum had constructed in 1887 special 'cottages' to house children separate to its adult inmate population. Part of the cottage complex included a schoolroom where the children were taught handwriting and gross-motor skills. But such an institution did not yet really exist in New South Wales. The Newcastle Hospital for the Insane housed one hundred children when it opened in 1871, but it wasn't until 1908 that a teacher was employed there to run classes.

William Taylor's parents, worried that he would set fire to their family home due to his 'mischievous' tenancies, had him committed to Callan Park in early December 1879. This boy, able to hear, but unable to speak or understand what was said to him, was diagnosed as having the 'vacant and unchanging expression of countenance of the [congenital] idiot'. Callan Park's first observation was William's lack of ability to 'attend to his own calls of nature' but it soon became clear that his major issue was his predisposition to the eating of pebbles at Callan Park when allowed into the airing courts – presumably of Ward One. After a liberal dose of castor oil, that favourite purgative of asylums at the time, on 17 December it was found that he had eaten fifteen ounces of rubbish. On 30 December, believing him to be free of pebbles, he was transferred to Newcastle Hospital where children were cared for. Record-keeping was not Newcastle's strong suit: it is alarming to read page after page of 'no change' recorded often for several years for the one patient. In addition, William's medical file recorded him wrongly as from Parramatta Asylum. His entries were brief and concise. In March, three months after his transfer there, he died, bleeding and in pain, from eating more pebbles.

Scholes managed the men at his hospital with great compassion and sympathy. By 1880 he had a much more substantial staff with which to do this. Besides Little, who continued as chief attendant, Scholes now had six male senior attendants, six junior attendants, a new outdoor attendant, John Cheetham, the son of the gardner, and an artisan attendant. Though the initial teething problems were numerous – unbalanced and unhappy patients, some of whom were aggressive, thrown together in small accommodation – Callan Park moved forward.

With Scholes' departure for Queensland came Callan Park's most notable superintendent, Dr Blaxland, the grandson of the famous explorer Gregory Blaxland. Soft featured and hair always strictly parted in all of his adult photos, Herbert Blaxland was born at the Hermitage at Ryde in 1852 to John and Ellen Blaxland. He attended the King's School, graduating from there in 1872.[35] After studying for two years at Sydney Hospital he went to London to study medicine.[36] When he returned to Australia, he returned as Dr Blaxland

and gained the post of assistant medical officer at Gladesville. From 1881, at twenty-nine years old, Callan Park became Blaxland's life. In 1882 he married Edith Jane Betts. He lived on site with her and his growing family: three sons, Guy (1883), Marcus (1884) the famous Queensland cricketer, and Faulkner (1886) and a daughter, Dorothy (1892), all born at Callan Park. He was medical superintendent there for nineteen years. His deputy was clerk Arthur Whitling, a keen photographer, and he captured numerous images of Blaxland's children growing up at Callan Park. Whitling's private family photo album[37] depicts Marcus Blaxland in particular. Blaxland's closeness with his staff, and particularly with Manning, is touching since through his career Blaxland was often Manning's chosen deputy – and there was certainly an element of master and apprentice in their collegiality and mutual respect. During his career, Blaxland was consistently made acting Inspector General, during Manning's occasional absences from the colony.[38]

Aside from being an avid and prize-winning horticulturist,[39] Blaxland was a passionate cricketer, often representing Callan Park or Gladesville alongside patients in inter-hospital competitions.[40] Manning's emphasis was on ornaments and pictures – and other homelike comforts – as leading to the cure of patients. Blaxland used sport in the same way: his patients were encouraged to play and be outside, breathing in the fresh air and stretching their legs. During his early tenure at Callan Park he had large amounts of fill removed from the grounds near Balmain Road so that a cricket pitch could be made[41], something which Frederick Legard made great use of. In the annual Inspector General *Reports* during Blaxland's time, he observed to Manning that the pitch was daily used by staff and patients, and that Callan Park often played Gladesville, the Orphan Schools, and various other institutions including the *Vernon*.[42] Blaxland implemented several other projects by which a boat house down near the water was erected, along with a garden shed in the kitchen garden for the storing of tools and to provide shelter for the patients when harvesting.[43] Blaxland's emphasis was on the outdoors, in patients working and relaxing outside in the sunshine. Under him, patients painted the weatherboard in order to maintain it, and the gardens were in a constant state of renovation and care;[44] Callan Park also became self sufficient for milk via its own cows on its farm.[45]

Blaxland occasionally bemoaned the difficulties of arranging amusements for such a small group of patients. When he arrived in 1881, Callan Park's population was at approximately 130 men. Cricket was a constant amusement, with regular matches on Saturdays something for patients to look forward to either as competitors or spectators – and practice during the week an excellent method of relaxation and distraction. There were fortnightly dances in the winter which patients attended at Gladesville since Callan Park's facilities did not yet include a hall where such an activity might be reasonably hosted. On Wednesdays patients were taken on tours of the harbour on the steam-launch, and picnics both at Gladesville and closer to home in Balmain were constant sources of interest and anticipation. Manning's desire that Sydney's own amusements be harnessed in the treatment of patients was also employed: Blaxland wrote in 1881[46] that select inmates heard 'the magnificent performances of the Australian Band', and visited the circus on a day trip at a later date. Performers also visited the hospital itself with dramatic and musical offerings: the Apollo Club, Balmain and Burwood Amateurs, the Balmain Coldstream Band and the Petersham Band all performed at Callan Park Hospital in its early days.

In 1882, Callan Park's church services – both Church of England and Roman Catholic – were given the addition of a harmonium, played by one of the new reverends' wives, Mrs Madgwick.[47] As a result, hymns were added to the services. In 1883 when Mr Russell took over the harmonium playing, a weekly choir practice was also added to the amusements of the week.[48] Legard's role in these is something which is unclear, but it is not unlikely that he was a knowledgeable assistant each Sunday.

While the patients sang, the contractors continued to work at Callan Park. The renovations at Garryowen, and Garryowen House itself, had only ever been a stopgap to deal with the immediate issue of ever-increasing lunatic numbers in the colony, and to provide relief to Gladesville in particular. But Garryowen was fast filling – and had never been the end-product anyway. Manning's monolithic hospital-proper, the Kirkbride Complex, set to house over 700 of the colony's insane, was beginning to take shape just a few metres away.

2

THE MENTAL STATE OF AUSTRALIA

To put it simply, there were too many lunatics in Australia.

In his first *Report* as Inspector of the Insane for the year 1876, Dr Frederic Norton Manning summarized that there had been an increase during the year of forty-three insane people in New South Wales, making a total of 1740 lunatics in the colony.[1] From 1864 to 1876 there had been an increase of 451, out of a population of about 500,000. This was too many for the asylums of the colony to cope with. Other states told the same story: in the same year, Victoria counted 2635 lunatics across its various asylums.[2]

There were a variety of reasons for this steady increase in numbers of patients over the 1860s and 1870s. Manning offered one point in particular – that more and more people were being certified as insane. He put this down to the 'growing intolerance on the part of the public... The vagrancies and eccentricities of this class are less and less borne with, and the attention of the police or other authorities more speedily directed to them than formerly... It appears certain that people are now considered and certified to be insane who would some twenty years ago have been held in a different estimation'.[3] The rise in medicine and healthcare was also accused as a promoter of the number of insane. Manning, in a paper on the *Causation and Prevention of Insanity* in 1880, wrote that '... our civilisation, in its varied and higher developments as well as in its manufacture of pauper and struggling classes, and especially in its many expedients for rendering possible, and prolonging the existence of those least fitted to survive and multiply, has caused and is still causing a higher percentage of insanity than was known in former times'.[4] In addition, Australia's position as a British colony on the opposite side of the world also made it a popular choice for relatives seeking to be rid of 'insane' family members, increasing the ratio in Australia of unwell to well. The numbers of mentally ill passengers arriving in Australia were a constant source of worry during these years, and a source of annoyance as they 'burdened' the colonies which in turn had to support them through the hospital system.[5]

Frederick Legard was one such patient.

Half a world away in the Yorkshire country side, and several decades before the Callan Park Asylum existed, Frederick Legard's parents met. Miss Cecilia Elizabeth Oldershaw knew very well that the reverend William Legard was a lunatic, but in 1803 she married him anyway.

William was the fourth son of the fifth Legard Baronet, whose seat was the tiny village of Ganton in North Yorkshire, England. In the late 1790s, when William was in his late twenties and early thirties, it was becoming clear that his family had a strong line of lunacy running through it. For William and his brothers, their childhood home of Ganton had become a veritable hothouse where their mad tendencies began to thrive with reckless abandon. William was first to slip: the wild child of his family, he was always keen to subvert his respectable Godly office via debauch and revelry. He was handed the living at Ganton's church, after his studies at Magdalen in Oxford were complete. The church at Ganton, St Nicholas, was made his – and instead of making his parish his first priority, William was distracted by a visitor to his neighbourhood.

William's brother Sir John was the inheritor of the baronetcy and grand Ganton Hall. Sometime around 1794 – when William had been presented his living at St Nicholas – Sir John made the decision to rent out Ganton Hall to the highest bidder rather than live in it himself. The man who moved in was called a 'wild, dissipated Irishman'[6] who has survived in the historical records only as 'Lord B'. This Lord B struck up an instant friendship with William who lived just down the road in the vicarage. William was young and, more importantly, prone to delight in excessive drinking. Such were the orgies up at the 'big house' that soon William was described as having suffered 'lasting injury to his constitution' as a result. His hard drinking had sparked a severe breakdown for which he was committed to an unknown asylum to recuperate.

William's family, thus left at little sleepy Ganton to contemplate the temporary loss of their brother, was struck with horror that their family name could be thus besmirched with the label of 'lunatic'. Such a name was dangerous in the 1700s and 1800s: it could cause family dishonour and drive a knife through the marriage and social aspirations of his siblings. But relief was quick: soon he was discharged, still needing support but able to work once more. The family was on edge: up until now William had seemed resilient, strong – if a little reckless – and it is quite reasonable to suppose that they wondered who else might yet bloom into insanity.

As William removed himself deliberately from Ganton, leaving his church in the hands of the local curate for some months, he installed himself in South Lincolnshire as a curate at Whaplode. His brother, Digby, and ever the 'fixer' of his family, stayed in Ganton to manage the affairs of the church and Hall. But now Digby had a new problem to deal with: the mania of Thomas, second in line to the Ganton fortune and brother to himself and William. Another mad brother was not exactly something to celebrate, but at least Thomas was not heir. But life has a way of twisting and turning, and soon Sir John was dead, having failed to produce an heir. His title and lands fell to the second brother: the lunatic Thomas. Digby was aghast.

Sir Thomas' lunacy was unlike William's, since its cause was not clear. In a letter dated 1797 from Digby to a family friend,[7] he described Thomas 'again being attacked as he was last year' with a peculiar type of lunacy: 'there is so much method in his madness that tis very difficult to determine whether tis insanity or not'. Digby felt the weight of such familial woe greatly, calling his brothers' illnesses the 'most horrible of maladies' and it being a burden almost too great to carry on the shoulders of the Legard family. Unlike William, Sir Thomas experienced many 'lucid intervals of considerable duration' which made it difficult to convince him he was ill, and even more so since 'unfortunately when he is in this forlorn way his best friends entirely loose [*sic*] their influence with him'. The family made a decision: the madhouse had done William a world of good, and so Thomas was carted off to follow in his footsteps. Thomas was soon installed at the luxurious Brooke House in London. His terror at his confinement is clear from a letter written in March 1797:[8] 'Surely,' he wrote, '... my relations can never think of my confining in a madhouse the remainder of my life[?]' and his pleading tone denotes his fear that his relatives, who he says never visited, might conveniently forget him. Later in his letter he makes an offer to quit England and be supported by a small salary of £120 – the same amount paid annually to Brooke House for his care – while his family repays his debts.

This offer was not accepted by the Legards who seem to have welcomed Sir Thomas home instead, as the mad baronet of Ganton Hall, to be managed at home rather than in a private establishment for the insane. When William brought his new wife, Cecilia Oldershaw, to the vicarage after their marriage in 1803, one can only wonder what her impression of the family was after her first visit to the Hall. Apparently unfazed – she *had* married an ex-madman after all – Cecilia and William got on with married life. Both excellent musicians, they had seven children together: three girls and four boys. Frederick Legard, the second youngest of the seven, was born on 23 October 1812 and was baptised a week later at Felixkirk in Yorkshire.[9]

By the time Frederick was born, Sir Thomas' issues had come to a head: he had been declared insane during an Inquisition in the Ganton Greyhound in 1811[10] and had been installed in the famous York Retreat, and was never released. William, on the other hand, continued well, and since Sir Thomas had been removed from society, so the shadow of madness lifted from the Legard family. Soon William – notably still slightly eccentric – was off again, leaving his wife to look after their then-six children alone. While his family stayed in Ganton, William began on an extraordinary solo adventure to Europe. Letters quoted by James Digby Legard RN, one of William's grandchildren, date his journey to 1815, when Frederick was but three years old. William asked often about his children, calling them Jem, Fred, Marianne, Bell, Harry and Willy, in his letters to his wife:

> *My little Frederick will be the flower of the flock and I hope will live to be the delight of his father. My poor Harriet will be steady in time, and Bell perhaps is too much at her age. Willy will make an honest man, and Jem a good farmer. Marianne will be a cocquette.*[11]

In many he makes special mention of Frederick, who appears ironically to have been the apple of his eye: 'Send my dear Fred in a box to me and I will send you back shawls, laces and stockings in abundance'.[12]

When he was eleven years old, in 1823, Frederick was sent away from Ganton and to school: to grand Charterhouse in Charterhouse Square, Smithfield, London. His brother James was beginning his own career in the British Navy by this time, and William Barnabas was ready to follow a similar path into the Army and the Sikh Wars in the future. But violence and war was not for William Legard's favourite son: Frederick was destined for the church and so began his education. He was nominated for a free scholarship by the Archbishop of Canterbury, who was a member of the governing body of Charterhouse, and Frederick was welcomed to the school as a 'Gownboy' thus named due to the wearing of an academic gown to denote his scholarly status at the school.

Legard's time at Charterhouse was one of great evolution[13] for the school, and one which he shared with William Makepeace Thackeray, who was in the year above him. Legard was installed at Charterhouse under the young headmaster Dr J. Russell, a man of a stern and angry disposition and a keen flogger of students, who implemented a range of changes to the institution. He lowered the price of education there by reducing the numbers of teachers. Instead, the school used the 'Madras' or 'Bell' system of education, where the older students or 'Præpositi' taught the younger. On occasion, these senior students – one hundred and twenty of them – were educated *en masse* by Dr Russell. In the early years of this system, which began when Legard was just beginning his schooling career, the number of enrolments at Charterhouse rose sharply. In 1818 there were a mere 238 boys at the school, and by 1825 – when Legard was in his third year there – 480 boys were at Charterhouse.

Dr Russell, meanwhile, disastrously did not increase the numbers of his staff and there were only eight masters to control almost 500 boys. Discipline was lax, the school became a magnet for students off ill-repute and bred more, and soon the school's reputation was in peril. Thackeray would come to parody its violence in his writings, calling it 'Slaughterhouse'.[14] In 1832, Legard's final year, Dr Russell and the Madras system was at an end, and the school population had plunged to a little over 100 students.

At school Legard's results were not spectacular,[15] but he moved up through the forms well. There was nothing to indicate any disturbance of mind or any ill health at this stage of his life, or any propensity to mimic his father or uncle. He was a normal teenager, and probably focused his energies on surviving Dr Russell's rough and violent institution. Even when in early 1826, when he was thirteen and away at school, his father died suddenly, still Legard attended classes regularly. This was a blow for both the Legards and Ganton. William was an important member of the baronet's family, being the fourth son of the fifth Legard Baronet. He had been baptised at Ganton's St Nicholas Church in 1765 and was the incumbent vicar. A handsome marble plaque was erected in the church to memorialise him, and is still there today. He was buried in the aisle of the church.

In 1832, after having lost his main support and role model in life, Frederick graduated from Charterhouse and entered Cambridge University. He was awarded an Exhibition to Emmanuel College, which indicated some merit in his final school results. Again, Legard moved through his university education at the normal speed, with a regular attendance and no bills for apothecaries on his Emmanuel account.[16] He studied mathematics and classics, and graduated with a BA in 1836. He left the university in 1838, being awarded an MA the following year. He graduated as a *Senior Optime,*[17] indicating a final result of second class honours in the *mathematical tripos*. By the time he was twenty-seven, Legard had a distinguished education behind him and he was ready to follow in the footsteps of his father in the clergy.

Immediately upon receipt of his MA he was ordained as a deacon by the bishop of Lincoln and in the following year Legard became a priest.[18] Soon, the Legard Baronets bestowed upon him the living at Ganton in North

Yorkshire, where his father have been reverend at the time of his death. Frederick Legard became the thirty-third vicar of Ganton.

Ganton is a tiny village about an hour by car out of York. On one side of the A64 is the Ganton Greyhound, the pub, and on the other is the village. Houses line the road – Main Street – up to the church and the vicarage – the currently standing one built in the 1850s after Frederick Legard's time. Wide open fields dominate the landscape, and pheasants, quietly cooing, are everywhere. The church itself sits high above the village on a little hill. It is small and dark inside, with light filtering in through the large stained glass windows, some of which have been dedicated to past reverends. The place is a mausoleum to the Legard family: marble plaques and funeral banners clutter the space and serve as a reminder of an ancient family long since decamped from the village. There is an original organ there, made electric some decades ago. Outside are graves, some hundreds of years old, along with new ones. Though St Nicholas has no vicar of its own these days, it is still a thriving church. Its clock still chimes out every hour as it would have during Frederick Legard's tenancy.

For the first four years, Legard found interest and purpose in his new career despite the death of the youngest of his siblings, Arthur, in 1842. Frederick was well-connected in Ganton: a cousin of the current Baronet, he would have enjoyed a healthy status in Ganton's small society. His elder brother James Anlaby was a successful captain in the Royal Navy. But most importantly, Frederick was returned to the place of his childhood, and transported back to the familiar surroundings he would have enjoyed as a boy with his father. In this period Legard's name was signed on all of the registers of St Nicholas Church, and it is clear he was an industrious vicar, even superintending renovation of the church during his early tenancy. But from 1846 the registers changed: curates' signatures amended documents relating to the church, and a large number, too. Legard's name was curiously absent and his church in the hands of a rotating roster of curates.[19]

The Legard family name was cast into darkness once more, but this time it was the small branch headed by matriarch Cecilia Legard which was affected, and not her wealthy baronet cousin's. Such a hereditary taint impacted on the family's standing in society and also in marriage prospects of both the sons and daughters; and from her subsequent actions, it is clear that Cecilia Legard feared the infamy which had accompanied Sir Thomas' committal would impact her own small brood. In January 1850 her second youngest child was committed to an asylum in Mansfield, called Broom House.[20] Her eldest son James Anlaby had just married, and was on the cusp of moving into his grand house at Kirby Misperton. Frederick, on the other hand, was exhibiting the same mental issues as her husband and brother-in-law had. It is unclear how Frederick Legard arrived in such a removed location from Ganton, and if he was committed by a family member or friend. The long distance between Ganton and Mansfield may indicate shame on the part of his family, and a wish to hide the details of his illness after the much-publicised case of Sir Thomas at the time of Frederick's birth. Records from Broom House, which was a private institution, do not survive today, and as a result it is impossible to know what Frederick was admitted for. It is tempting to wonder if he was showing symptoms similar to those of his uncle, Sir Thomas. Broom House catered for both men and women, in discreetly separate sections. Legard was admitted as a private patient to the large manor house, under the care of a Dr Wilson, whose mad-house was problematically located next door to the Mansfield railway station. In the UK *Lunacy Register* Legard is recorded, in minute and rather abashed handwriting, as having 'escaped and returned' at some point in 1850. Legard was used to institutions, having been a member of the rough Charterhouse as a child: surviving such a place was in his blood. By the middle of August he was discharged as recovered.

But Legard was not entirely cured and it is possible that his family removed him from care, after his successful escape, despite the fact he was not well – as had been the case for a time with Sir Thomas. Frederick returned to Ganton and continued in his role as reverend there, administering his parish with the assistance of a band of visiting curates and vicars of neighbouring parishes. In 1851 his sister Isabel and her husband William Chester were living in the vicarage, presumably caring for him.[21] Legard continued unmarried and suddenly in 1852 resigned his position as vicar of Ganton due to 'ill health'.[22] He was quickly replaced by Disney Legard Alexander, a distant relative.

Cecilia Legard was not happy with this turn of events. A rather wealthy widow, she was used to having her way. At the same time that Frederick was taken to Broom House she decided to write her will.[23] Her primary aim was that her daughters would not be left to any unfortunate fate or be dependent upon the men in their family for charitable handouts after her death. Her eldest son, James Anlaby, was to receive his land and monies upon her decease, but was required to support via rents and the rest his three sisters – particularly Mary Anne and Henrietta who were both unmarried – to assure them of their comfort. Not until the last of his three sisters were dead, would James be able to keep the income generated by his immense property and would his brothers, William Barnabas and Frederick, receive a penny. Frederick's future annuity was listed as amounting to £40 per year, paid from James Anlaby's estate. William Barnabas was to receive a much more generous lump sum of £4,000. Cecilia appears to have had the shame and scandal of Broom House at the forefront of her mind when she put pen to paper.

Out of work and in the stages of recovery, it is unclear what Legard was doing for the next five years. At the end of 1854 his mother was dead. By this time James was installed in his new home at Kirby Misperton and for a time played host to William Barnabas' wife and child while he fought in the Sikh Wars.[24] It is possible that James offered Frederick a place to stay during his recuperation.

In 1857 Legard dropped off the list of English Clergy and packed up his life in England and booked passage to Australia, in a move reminiscent of his father's European jaunt after his own recovery. Frederick Legard arrived in Sydney in January 1858, apparently well. Why this sudden decision to move, is unclear. The thought of a new life, away from the stresses – or triggers – of his ill health, may have been appealing. Equally possible is that his family, already tainted by Sir Thomas' madness, sought to relieve the family name by shipping him off to one of the colonies in a move familiar to the tax payers of Australia.

Australia's mental health care at this time was very different to the lunatic landscape in England. England's system of care consisted of two distinct arms – the public and private spheres. There were state institutions which cared for criminal lunatics and ex-military men, and there were wards in poor houses for paupers. Famous institutions such as Bedlam were of this kind. These were run by various levels of country and district governance. But there were also thriving private institutions, such as the famous Ticehurst in Sussex where John Perceval was housed, and Broom House where Legard was sent, where patients of more disposable means could be cared for in smaller groups, sometimes singly. These, as can be imagined, varied in quality and purpose. Many of the Lunacy Act amendments in Britain at this time were to counter the shady practices of various ill-qualified or ill-intentioned 'mad-doctors' or alienists, as they were called.

In Australia, however, the circumstances were quite different, a situation observed by Dr Manning. Private institutions were virtually unheard of in this time in both New South Wales and Victoria. The only one in New South Wales was Bayview House, near Cook's River at Tempe. Like Garryowen, Bayview had once been a private home and was converted to an asylum by the addition of weatherboard buildings to the sides of the house which by 1880 were regarded as old and fitted with rather antiquated appliances.[25] The first patient was admitted in November 1865 under the care of Dr George A. Tucker, who had been previously a managing partner at various other Melbournian asylums.[26] Cook's River could accommodate only a small number and was quite unpopular[27] ; thus the bulk of the burden of caring for the mentally ill fell to the state in New South Wales and Victoria, with little relief from private enterprise.

New South Wales was, and had been from the beginning of European settlement, the leader amongst the Australian colonies in terms of mental health. For one, Queensland and Tasmania for some time depended upon the transfer of patients to New South Wales for its residents' care, not having any institution of their own. For another, New South Wales' Tarban Creek Asylum (later Gladesville Asylum) was the mother institution of Victoria's Yarra Bend, that state's first mad-house.

The Tarban Creek Asylum was the first purpose-built hospital[28] for the treatment of the insane on the Australian mainland, and was opened in 1838 in Gladesville, a suburb of Sydney in New South Wales. Its sprawling sandstone buildings still stand today beside busy Victoria Road. Its existence was borne out of the need for a dedicated and extensive institution for the care of the growing number of lunatics in the state after the closure of Castle Hill Asylum. Castle Hill, also in Sydney, was opened in 1811 but the cramped conditions and lack of staff caused its closure and transfer of patients to the Liverpool Court House less than two decades later in 1825. Patients remained in the court house until Tarban Creek was built. But Tarban Creek was by no means perfect, and the patients awaiting it would have been rather underwhelmed. In 1863, Dr Wilson, the Catholic bishop of Hobartown at the time, wrote to the Colonial Secretary,[29] labelling the buildings at Gladesville 'ill-constructed', 'gloomy', and severely lacking in facilities such as a hall – for amusements and chapel services – a farm or yards for exercise. At the time, these were increasingly seen as compulsory elements of any worthwhile asylum. He scorned the poor choice of situation – which was rather isolated, impacting the visitation of patients' relatives and friends, and also the ease with which deliveries of supplies might be made – as well as the lack of 'classification' of patients, according to their different symptoms and treatment. Patients suffering melancholia were housed with those of a more maniacal disposition, creating disharmony in the wards and in the process hindering treatment. Henry Parkes agreed with him, calling Gladesville 'an unsightly prison' with locks on every door, bars on every window and a denial of outdoor exercise for patients. 'It was the principal asylum of the country,' Parkes would come to admit, 'and the unfortunate inmates were kept in a worse condition than prisoners, having no exercise, and with no single influence arising from objects of beauty to alleviate their dark and dismal condition'.[30]

To alleviate the over-crowding at Tarban Creek, Parramatta Asylum was opened in 1849. This was a common system in nineteenth century Australia: one asylum spawned another. The same had occurred in Melbourne with Yarra Bend: after having cut apron strings from Tarban Creek in 1851 – where it became Yarra Bend Asylum, rather than Yarra Bend, Branch Establishment of Tarban Creek – Yarra Bend came to produce Kew Asylum, in an attempt to deal with the constant influx of more insane, in 1871. At Parramatta the building was not new, as with Tarban Creek, but a converted factory prison. Similar issues arose here: the iron barred doors and the cell-like rooms[31] were not conducive to the treatment of mental illness in the slightest. In contrast to Tarban Creek though, Parramatta's use was two-fold: to lessen the burden on Tarban Creek as the main receiving hospital in the state for lunatics, and also to securely house the criminally insane and act as a branch of Parramatta Gaol. Parramatta Asylum catered for both types of insane criminals: those who while insane committed crimes, and also those who became insane while serving their sentences.[32]

With this increase in provisions for the mentally unwell, Henry Parkes found himself in a quandary in the 1860s. New South Wales had two asylums in Tarban Creek and Parramatta, and one small private asylum at Cook's River, but no energetic regulator of these. He wanted a medical doctor, and a humane one too, to superintend these institutions – someone who could steer his state's asylums into the realm of quality and safety, and create for New South Wales the premier asylums of Australia. In Dr Frederic Norton Manning he found such a man.

Parkes had seen what was occurring in Victoria's state asylums and wished to avoid the same controversy in New South Wales. Victoria's asylum system was younger than New South Wales' and yet in the 1860s and 1870s was already a source of suspicion and unrest for the state. In 1876 the fear came to a head in the form a series of six articles appeared in the *Argus* entitled 'A Month in Kew Asylum and Yarra Bend'.[33] The journalist responsible for the series, who used the apt pseudonym 'Vagabond' to disguise his identity, had gone undercover and worked in two of the state's asylums as an attendant. His object was to throw light onto the reprehensible conduct of asylum staff, and the conditions patients were forced to endure. His articles do not make for comfortable reading. Vagabond wrote of the under-training of staff – as a new attendant with no experience being made to work with high-dependency and violent patients in the Hospital Wards – and the poor conditions where staff were vastly outnumbered by patients and forced to rely on the assistance of the mad to ensure the working of the institution. Cramped conditions, where day rooms where conscripted as bedrooms, with beds crushed in side by side, and the disparity of staff salaries – indicated as a reducer of morale among attendants – were graphically recorded. Violence to patients was a starring element of Vagabond's prose, giving details of the general abuse of patients by staff – in teasing the blind, for instance, by giving them false names by which to report their ill-discipline – and unnecessary force. He described the 'simplification' of an attendant's duties by 'passing one's arm round a patient's throat *à la garrotte*, and lifting him by the chin, dragging or pushing him' and the way to 'encourage' a patient: 'by a 'clout' on the side of the ear – that is a blow given with full force with the flat of the hand. It will not mark, but will certainly pain'. In describing the workings of the Hospital Ward, Vagabond described the primary work: to 'keep a look out for epileptics. When these latter get a fit, the simple way is just to pull them on the floor, see that they are unconfined at the neck, and let them have it out. Now and then a blind man may walk on to them, which only makes it more amusing'. Questions about discipline, particularly from the superintendent, were dealt with easily: Vagabond recorded the man on his rounds asking tokenistically 'All well here?' and the answer always being a positive one.

Parkes did not want the same situation in New South Wales as Victoria was struggling under, and Manning was the perfect antidote. Manning was born in Rothershorp in Northamptonshire on 25 February 1839. After studying medicine at St George's Hospital, England, he became a member of the Royal College of Surgeons at the age of twenty-one. A slight man of middle height, with his high collar and necktie, he was the very picture of a Victorian gentleman. In all of his portraits he is shown as balding, and with the same intelligent, but sensitive, look in his eye. Always interested in international goings-on, he soon after joined the Royal Navy as a surgeon on HMS *Esk*. Aboard *Esk* he saw considerable active service and was present in New Zealand for much of the Maori War. During the first attack on Gate Pah at Tauranga, where the British were unsuccessful, an injured man whom Manning was endeavouring to carry to safety was shot through the heart as he held him.[34] Still a surgeon in the Navy, in 1867 Manning arrived in Sydney and was met by Parkes, who 'became convinced that he was the sort of man which the government wanted in carrying out a thorough reform in [the] methods of treatment, and [he] proposed to [Manning] that he should obtain his discharge from the service to which he was then attached, and accept the principal office in [the] department of lunacy. This he assented to'.[35]

Manning was made medical superintendent of New South Wales' primary asylum, Tarban Creek (which came to be known as Gladesville Hospital), in November that year. Victoria had a similar idea and appointed its first, and one might say fairly lacklustre, Inspector of Lunatic Asylums and Licensed Houses, Dr Edward Paley, medical superintendent of Yarra Bend, also in 1867. But right from the beginning, Paley was outclassed by Manning. One of the latter's first, and almost immediate, reforms was to change the name of this Gladesville institution from 'Tarban Creek Asylum' to 'Hospital for the Insane, Tarban Creek' and then 'Hospital for the Insane, Gladesville'. This was an important distinction for Manning – that between 'asylum' and 'hospital' – who called it

> *... A trifling matter it may seem; but trifles go far to make up the sum of human happiness everywhere, and are magnified a thousand-fold in the atmosphere of an Institution of this character ... I have no fault to find with the word asylum, it is a good enough word in itself, but it means something more than a refuge. It suggests a permanent abiding place, and has become surrounded with sad and sombre associations. It rings a knell in the ears of many a patient, whereas the word hospital suggests hope, cure, and restoration. Besides, too, a deep truth underlines the change: it is the difference between a cemetery for disordered intellect and a hospital for diseased brains.*[36]

Aside from this subtle change in language, Manning had a further point to make: his institution was a *hospital*. It was headed by medical men with a team of medical officers supporting them, not gaolers or wardens as in the old days of the early colony. The records for Callan Park's early years make clear the amount of medical assistance occurring in these institutions. In 1883, a patient who was involved in a scuffle with another was obliged to wait until the medical superintendent returned to reduce a dislocation of the shoulder.[37] Amputations were also conducted, regular vaccinations of patients carried out; patients who were bleeding were stitched up, and even one emergency tracheotomy was performed.[38] Manning also advocated for the replacement of the term 'lunatic' with 'insane', the former being 'from a popular belief in influences [of the moon] that have long since been shown to have no existence'.[39]

The following year, Parkes commissioned Manning to 'visit Europe and America to enquire into, and report upon, the whole subject of the care and management of the insane as illustrated by the plans of construction, economic arrangements, and systems of treatment, in the best-known asylums'.[40] Manning visited asylums in Britain, including famous institutions such as Broadmoor and Bedlam, along with hospitals in America and Europe. His findings were produced in a book, *Report on Lunatic Asylums,* which came to be regarded as a 'standard work',[41] and many of his ideas, sourced from his tour, were faithfully reproduced at both Gladesville and Callan Park. The gap between Manning's New South Wales institutions and Paley's in Victoria continued to widen.

In 1876, the same year Callan Park received its first patients, Legard among them, Manning became the Inspector of the Insane, and continued to superintend Gladesville Hospital. On the passing of the 1878 Lunacy Act, he became the Inspector General of the Insane and was obliged to resign his position at Gladesville in order to successfully oversee the care of patients not just there, but throughout the entire state. As Inspector General, Manning was responsible for drafting the relevant legislation for the various Lunacy Acts, and ensuring that facilities and treatment used in New South Wales' asylums were on par with those in the rest of the world – particularly Britain and America. The office also required him to petition the Colonial Secretary for funds for improvements and facilities, and to ensure New South Wales' laws were upheld in New South Wales' asylums. He also made frequent visits to Gladesville, Parramatta, Cook's River and Callan Park to ensure patient safety, the standards of cleanliness, food and care. Dealing with complaints – from patients, staff, relatives of patients – were also in his domain.

The New South Wales Lunacy Department was run transparently, and with strict adherence to the laws it helped to write.[42] When Manning took charge, the state was running on the basis of the 1843 Dangerous Lunatics Act, which was based on the 1828 English Act of the same name. It required two doctors to certify the status of a man or woman's lunacy and appointed visitors to the state's asylums who reported back to the Colonial Secretary. Manning's 1867 Lunacy Act amended the 1843 Act by the introduction of a Reception House for the insane – namely, a high-turnover processing hospital where lunatics were sent pending admittance to a hospital such as Gladesville or Parramatta. Now, medical certificates were required to contain the facts the diagnosis was based upon – rather than a mere diagnosis and two doctors' signatures – to safeguard against wrongful admission, and hospitals for the insane were obliged to keep accurate records of patients' medical treatment, admittance and discharge.

These changes, and tightening of procedure, reflected the community's fear of wrongful admittance to asylums. On numerous occasions Manning spoke directly to this fear, repeating in several of his *Reports* his close attention to all cases of lunacy and his strict examination of all warrants and petitions.[43] In 1882 he found reason to reject a medical certificate on the grounds that it was signed by an unqualified practitioner[44] and in 1886 liberated a patient admitted to Parramatta and diagnosed him as suffering from acute delirium caused by typhoid fever rather than insanity.[45] Rules prohibiting the 'sequestration of persons who are sane, for improper purposes'[46] included the voiding of certificates signed by father and son, two medical partners or a practitioner and his assistant, or a medical superintendent of any asylum. The 1878 Lunacy Act, written by Manning, reiterated many of these elements and created the office of Inspector General. It also expanded the number records to be kept by hospitals and created the office of master-in-lunacy, part of the Supreme Court, which dealt with the property of lunatics.

With Manning's arrival in New South Wales came a new era in the treatment of mental illness. Never before had the asylums had such a united leadership – and one based in medical knowledge and benevolence. After arriving in New South Wales, he grew the state's asylum care from two to six major hospitals, and he regulated the admissions system and ruled his department with fairness and sympathy. In turn, Manning became a world authority on the treatment of mental illness, lecturing at Sydney University. He was elected as the president of the Board of Health and was for a time a medical advisor to the government, besides being a trustee of the National Art Gallery.[47] He devoted his life to his patients, remaining unmarried his entire life, and without family in Australia. When he died in 1903, five years after retiring from his position of Inspector General, and at the age of sixty-four, his coffin was met by sixty attendants from the hospitals he had designed and watched over. When his coffin was lowered into the ground, on the edge of Gladesville Asylum – a gesture which was not lost on the patients and staff who were mourners at the ceremony – it was recorded that the flags fluttering over the ferry boats floating nearby were all at half-mast.[48]

The situation in Victoria was vastly different. While the care of lunatics in New South Wales expanded and buoyed under Manning, Victoria's state system was in dire need of review, drowning under the influence of a motley assembly of stand-in Inspectors after Paley's resignation in 1883. In 1886 a Royal Commission, the 'Zox' Commission,[49] was launched to investigate that state's hospitals for the insane and inebriate. Zox's recommendations were comprehensive and took much from New South Wales' organisation. Among the points presented were that the classification of patients – particularly those who were criminal – ought to be increased, and that provision ought to be made for patients of higher classes in paying wards. Dangerous patients were suggested to be housed away from those of a more predictable character, and patients should not be committed indefinitely. Importantly, it was argued that the power of discharge be transferred to the hands of the medical superintendent 'without other authority'.

As Victoria floundered, New South Wales advanced. Manning's were 'hospital[s] where care and skills are employed in the treatment of those most to be pitied on this earth; not, as is now too often the case, as a prison in which beings, little better than wild beasts, are shut from the gaze of mankind'.[50] But the lunatic population was still an issue. As Inspector General of the Insane, Manning would have been painfully aware of the overcrowding across all of the asylums in New South Wales in the 1870s. The obvious solution for the lack of accommodation for New South Wales' insane was to extend Gladesville into a larger institution, but Manning did not advocate this. Its isolation, and the consequent extra expense incurred by building there,[51] made the site undesirable for Manning's revolution. Parramatta was also not ideal:

> *After special and close examination of Parramatta and* [Gladesville] – *both before and since an inspection of the asylums of Europe and America – the conclusion has been arrived at, that the buildings at Parramatta are utterly and completely unfit for the purpose for which they are at present employed ... In such buildings the proper care and treatment of the insane is simply impossible ... with its gloomy, ill-ventilated cells, with their iron-barred doors ... The new building for criminals seems to have been built solely with a view to the safe keeping of its inmates – a prison within an asylum... and differs, in almost every particular, from the buildings used as hospitals for insane criminals at Broadmoor, Perth,* [England] *and Auburn, U.S. ... Notwithstanding the beautiful views to be obtained from* [Gladesville], *it is, from its inherent structure, the smallness of its windows, the confined nature of its airing courts... extremely gloomy and prison-like ...*[52]

Manning cited two experts from an 1863 report, Dr Wilson and Dr Boyd, who each[53] suggested a site closer to the city of Sydney being the best choice. Manning concurred with Dr Wilson's arguments concerning Sydney as the ideal location: that Sydney's central location would attract the best medical men and attendants, and provide the best amusements for patient outings.[54]

Manning's vision[55] was set: Gladesville would continue with 300 patients, the new Sydney asylum with 500, Parramatta would be exclusively for the criminally insane and house up to 80 – and three new 'up country' asylums at Goulburn, Bathurst and Maitland, holding 600 in total, would be established – thus accommodating 1,480 patients across New South Wales. Though Manning's plan was not fully realised – Parramatta continued to hold 'ordinary' patients, and the 'up country' hospitals were not put into action for a few decades more – the jewel in his crown – the establishment of a large hospital for the insane in Sydney – was. But the first step was acquiring the land.

At some point in the 1840s, when Frederick Legard was making his sermons in Ganton, John Ryan Brenan built Garryowen House. It was a private residence surrounded by an immense park, and Brenan used it as his own home. The layout of the mansion lent itself wonderfully towards parties, and even boasted a ballroom. Its lavishness is still clear today with its ornate floating staircase and beautiful window frames. In 1865 the estate was bought by business man John Gordon, who named the entire estate Callan Park after the River Callan which ran past his Irish home,[56] and renamed Garryowen 'Callan Park House'. Curiously, even to this day, this name will not stick. Ever the businessman, in 1873 Gordon decided to sell Garryowen and divide the rest of Callan Park, some eighty-one acres, into sixty-seven 'villa sites' or lots, also for sale.[57] Henry Parkes, in consultation with Manning and the Colonial Architect James Barnet, snapped up the entire property for a mere £65,000, an action of which he boasted on more than one occasion in parliament.[58] The keys to Garryowen were handed to the government in July 1874.[59]

With Manning at the helm, New South Wales' mad seemed in good hands. His attention to detail, energy, and conviction that everything must be done by the book, meant that the Lunacy Department was run smoothly. But paperwork and statistics do not a hospital make: it is the staff and the conditions upon which such institutions are judged. Charles Reade and John Perceval had not just *imagined* the poor treatment of the insane, and it was alive and well even in Sydney.

3

THE KIRKBRIDE COMPLEX

Whatever the reason, Legard enjoyed many years of fine health as a result of his removal from England. If he suffered from the same disease as his uncle Sir Thomas, he was experiencing a 'lucid interval' of several years' duration. He lived in style in Brighton Park in Melbourne. Brighton Park, today the beach-front suburb bounded by the Esplanade, and Wellington and Park Streets, was a sought-after address in the 1850s. The land was originally bought and lived in by Henry Dendy in the 1840s. Failing as a business man, he was declared insolvent and in 1848 the land was sold and eventually divided into lots, presided over by an immense manor house and Church of England church. By 1854 it was billed as the 'celebrated Brighton Estate'.[1] Legard's name and address would have bought him friends in his new home of Melbourne; his intelligence would have further recommended him. Unlike so many foreigners who found in Australia isolation and sunstroke and thus insanity, Legard's mental balance seems to have been soothed by his removal from friends and family.

In June 1858, three and a half years after the death of his mother, he had a letter to the editor of *The Age* published, 'The Railway Aspect',[2] a document which demonstrated his knowledge of the world and his learning. At this time, he was clearly of sound mind: his expression is clear and lucid. He wrote, 'Sir, – As we appear to be on the eve of a railway era, perhaps it may not be amiss to take a prospective view of what we are about. Looking upon our railway system, then, in a military, social, and commercial point of view ...' Legard's letter went into some detail and offered various solutions for a united Australia connected by railway tracks. He wrote on:

> … *We should have a connection with a line of floating steam batteries, (plying constantly between Adelaide, Melbourne, and Sydney, and used in time of peace for commercial purposes,) a pretty complete system of coast-guard defence, whereby the united force of the confederate States of Australia might be readily concentrated upon any threatened point of attack. Besides the military view of the case, the same would form a famous base line in a commercial point of view … But I would not stop here, for I don't see why the United States Government of Australia, in connection with the imperial home of Government, could not form a line from the Upper Darling to the Albert River, at the head of the Gulf of Carpentaria.* [He concluded with:] *This would at once afford a complete solution of the questions – how are we to meet the over-immigration of the Chinese? and what is to be done with the Sepoys? For by forming Sepoy, Malay and Chinese settlements along with line in the tropical regions of North Australia, where they could cultivate their native products, under the British rule, an extensive market for Eastern goods might be established within our own territories … We should make Melbourne and these colonies the centre of the immense traffic of the south-eastern basin of the globe, and the British Empire the commercial mistress of the world. Thus, as railways produce union, and union produces strength, so likewise … we might by these means fulfil a far higher destiny, and promote the end of prosperity, strength, and peace.*

Legard was well. He was productive and, to quote the terminology used routinely at Callan Park, 'able to look after himself'. It is unclear how he was supporting himself, but it is likely that his savings from his decade as a priest would have been at his disposal, and if his family had really chosen to be rid of him and shipped him off to Australia, it is possible that some kind of allowance had been given to him.

But then Legard briefly left his comfortable existence in Australia. Perhaps the lack of support he received at Broom House was indicative of a rift between himself and his family, mitigated by his sister Isabel and her husband, and he felt that time and distance had now healed the wounds. The familial discomfort endured by Legard is best depicted through the situation of his mother's will. The animosity emanating from his mother was made clear in her division of her property and wealth. Legard, though a beneficiary, was to receive the least of his brothers and sisters by a long way, and this cannot have gone unnoticed by her youngest son. The fact that Cecilia's mean bequest was made one month after Legard's release from Broom House in 1850 is also quite telling.

But the exact purpose of Legard's costly visit to England at this time is unknown – the date does not coincide with any major family event other than the death of William Chester, Isabel's husband, in 1858, who had lived in the vicarage with Legard during his recuperation – and was a short one, since he arrived back in Sydney in early 1859. Legard's siblings were all still alive in England at this point, but it is unknown if he even met with them. It is possible he went to offer his condolences to Isabel, and to visit his new nieces and nephews, as both James and Isabel had families of their own by this time. It is also possible that he went to discuss the possible sale of some property jointly owned by himself and his siblings. The property was in Loughborough and consisted of a farmhouse, plantation and several acres of land. Legard's siblings sold their shares in this to a W. P. Herrick in April 1859.[3] In 1861, and possibly indicative of his dwindling wealth, Legard was returned to Melbourne, from where he sold his interest in his family's estate at Loughborough in England to the same W. P. Herrick.[4]

Lacking both occupation and a regular income, Legard became a teacher in 1864. An advertisement in the *Argus* ran thus:

VICTORIAN COLLEGIATE INSTITUTION.
(Le Bignell's Hotel)
Principal – the Rev K M MYERS.
PROFESSORS
Classics and Mathematics – Frederic [sic] *Legard, Esq., senior optime and MA of Cambridge University.*

French – Mons. D'Aloustel, University Paris.
Elocution – T P Bill, Esq
Natural Sciences – Dr Macadam
School duties will recommence (DV) pm Monday January 4.[5]

Legard had a job, and one which acknowledged his university education – with Rev Meyers headlining the advertisement for his school with Legard's qualifications – and yet in February 1865 he left Melbourne for England again, this time on the *True Briton.* Again, the visit was short, with Legard returning to Victoria the following year on the SS *Great Britain*, a grand and innovative ship which was possibly one of the world's first ocean liners. Why this costly visit was made by Legard and for what purpose is again unclear.

Legard's return to his adopted home state of Victoria was also short: in 1867 he moved to Sydney where he found more teaching work at Mademoiselle Naegueli's Boarding and Day School, where he taught English 'daily'. But now, oddly, he was 'Mr Legard, BA' only.[6] Perhaps his increasingly erratic nature lost his job for him, or his eccentricities made him leave of his own accord – but soon Legard was not teaching anymore. For the next two years he still supported himself, his savings all but used up, writing letters and keeping books for tradesmen, but his position in society was deeply at odds with that which he had previously enjoyed. Legard began exhibiting the classic signs of one in mental distress, and began on a path which would lead him to Callan Park.

As in the outside world, work was an important element of life at Callan Park.

Manning, along with many of his Victorian colleagues in the south, was a great believer in Moral Therapy as being the key to the treatment of the insane. Moral Therapy was built upon several principles, the most prominent being the inclusion of kindness in the management of lunatics. Compassion and sympathy meant that sufferers would be treated as human beings and patients, rather than inmates and animals. Interwoven into this humane attitude was a respect of patients, and the acknowledgment of their skills and interests. As such, work held an important status in any institution aligned with Moral Therapy: it was encouraged as part of the rehabilitation process, a perfect distraction to the stresses and unhappiness of an unsound mind. But work – both the ability to be useful, and more importantly the *desire* to be occupied – was also seen as a sign of cure or at least a large step made on the road to recovery. In 1895 Blaxland was interviewed by the *Sunday Times*, which recorded his thoughts on this topic:

> *No compulsory service is extracted from the patients, but those in a fit state of bodily and mental health are generally only too anxious for occupation. In fact, as Dr. Blaxland says, it is the best medicine for the mentally diseased, and one of the best signs of convalescence is when the inmates begin to enquire of something to do.*[7]

Hospitals such as Callan Park were well-equipped with places to work: farms, workshops for painting and carpentry, engine rooms, and the kitchen and laundry. The work was real work: patients made furniture, completed renovations of the buildings and gardens, and as such none was done on a Sunday,[8] a strong indication that at Callan Park the patients were not enlisted into work as slaves of the attendants, as Vagabond[9] implied was occurring in Victoria's asylums. Any fears of unwell patients misusing tools were unfounded, according to Manning:

> *With a proper selection of occupation for the various classes of patients, little danger is to be apprehended from entrusting patients with tools and implements. Accidents from this cause are very few in asylums, and to run some small risk, and so benefit the great mass of patients, is undoubtedly better than to prevent work for fear of accidents.* [And besides ...] *The patients supported at the expense of the State may fairly be expected to work for its benefit.*[10]

Moral Therapy had further ideals: patients were to be treated kindly and, where possibly, without the use of mechanical restraint. Such restraints included camisoles and straightjackets – with the sleeves sewn into the pockets. Also used were muffs – which were leather gloves fastened together and with the ability to be locked and could be used to prevent suicide, mischief with dressings or bandages as the result of some treatment, and masturbation. Lastly, restraint also included seclusion in padded rooms or, as at Garryowen, possibly in the basement below the entrance hall. These modes of restraint were used at Callan Park, but certainly not routinely. Any application of any kind of restraint was recorded and subject to approval by Manning as Inspector General of the Insane. Manning also required such mechanisms were 'to be used only by the direct order of one of the Medical Officers ... [and] it is distinctly understood that they are, when not in use, to be kept under lock and key by one of the officers, and not accessible to the attendants and nurses'.[11] In a typical week at Callan Park only two or three patients might be expected to have been restrained with camisoles or muffs; no more than this were secluded. Of course, some weeks saw nil for both. The small numbers of patients requiring such assistance – tallies difficult to fake unless Manning and staff at Callan Park were colluding each week for many decades – demonstrate that these methods were a last resort and certainly not the norm.

Callan Park's arsenal in terms of restraint was limited to these means and appears to have been a remarkably transparent process. The medical records always provide a reason for any restraint. But here we have a possible smudge on the record of Callan Park with the existence of an article from W. L. Lindsay in the *American Journal of Insanity* in 1878,[12] claiming Manning's interest in a restraint called the 'Utica Crib' or 'Protection Bed' which Lindsay had invented. The Protection Bed was a horrific wooden cage containing a sleeping pallet which locked from the outside and which was advertised as a way to 'protect' the patient thus within from self-harm. In his article, Lindsay wrote that:

> *At his* [Manning's] *instigation that government of that colony applied to me, in February, 1879, for a specimen of the protection beds actually used in the Murray Royal Institution, Perth* [in Scotland], *and the result was, that one was at once supplied for*

> *the purpose of transmission to Sydney, and of introduction into the public asylums of New South Wales.*

There is, however, absolutely nothing to suggest that Manning actually promoted the use of this contraption in his hospitals. There is no mention of it in patient notes and if George Morton had been in one, he would no doubt have included such in his writing. To say that Lindsay was lying is a rather large call to make, but a closer look at the article in question provides a possible rationale to this odd smear on Manning and his hospitals. Lindsay's article refers to Manning as unparalleled in the civilised world in terms of his knowledge of insanity. It is possible that the entire article is an extended advertisement, using Manning unwittingly as an endorsement.

Thus patients were to be outside, exercising, being stimulated – most importantly – in beautiful places. It was pivotal that the environment and buildings be aesthetically pleasing, unlike the gloomy and depressing Parramatta and Gladesville which would eventually be renovated to match Manning's Moral Therapeutic aims. It was with these stipulations in mind that Manning's Callan Park proper began its construction, just a little removed from Garryowen House and its weatherboard extensions. James Barnet, the Colonial Architect, had designed the buildings with Moral Therapy in mind: a series of pavilion-style blocks in the rough design of the Kirkbride pattern, named after the famous American Moral Therapist Dr Thomas Story Kirkbride. Dr Kirkbride's enlightened design was used throughout America and Europe and at the time was regarded as the blueprint for successful treatment of the insane, as the architecture was thought to allow best for the principles of Moral Therapy to be put into action: outdoor spaces, light and airy rooms, short corridors, and the separation of patients to minimise disturbances and increase privacy. For Barnet this meant that the hospital would be clean and hygienic, something which he saw as paramount after a visit to Gladesville Hospital in the days prior to Manning's arrival in the colony:

> [He] *said that about 20 years ago* [before Manning had arrived in the colony] *he paid his first official visit to ... Tarban Creek. Then*

he saw such sights as he hoped never to see again, and they affected him so that he was unable to sleep for three nights afterwards. The rats were running over the patients, the gutters were stinking, the closets overflowing, and everything was in a fearful condition. He resolved, that if ever he got a chance, he would do what he could to make better provision for the poor people, and build a new lunatic asylum.[13]

Many Kirkbride buildings exist today: St Elisabeth's in Washington DC and New Jersey State Hospital at Trenton, New Jersey, are but two fine examples. Barnet's design differed slightly from the traditional Kirkbride plan in that Callan Park's pavilions were separate buildings rather than staggered wings of a single building. Technically therefore not an authentic Kirkbride, the new Callan Park asylum building, known today as the Kirkbride Complex, was clearly *inspired* by the famous design.[14]

If the new Callan Park was not technically a Kirkbride, it was certainly a Nightingale. In 1868 Manning wrote that 'the principles of hospital construction which have been laid down by Miss Nightingale ... [apply] to hospitals for mental diseases'.[15] By this he referred to Nightingale's 'Environmental Theory' which emphasized the importance of cleanliness, light and air for the treatment of the ill. Chartham Asylum in Kent was Callan Park's model, with the addition of verandahs and outdoor spaces to 'meet the requirements of the climate of New South Wales'.[16]

Of course, there were delays to the beginning of the Kirkbride Complex's construction. In 1877 the *Sydney Morning Herald* pointed out that the use of Garryowen as an asylum was only ever to be a temporary measure while the state awaited the completion of the new buildings which were to be the hospital-proper. 'A site was purchased at Callan Park for a new building, £75,000 voted towards its erection four years ago, and yet nothing has been done. For what does the Executive exist but to carry out the work which Parliament has decided to have done?'[17] But in 1880 the contract was won by Messers Low and Kerr,[18] with the ground broken on 11 February 1880. The construction was steady from then on. In April 1883, a year and a half out from the final completion of the work, and only two months before its originally-promised completion date,[19] one of the cornerstones of the water tower was ceremonially laid:

> *Mr James Barnet, Colonial Architect, was invited to perform the ceremony. The stone was lowered into position about half-past three. In a cavity beneath it was placed a bottle containing copies of the daily newspapers published in the city, some current coins of the realm, and a scroll setting forth the dates of the laying of the first stone and of the present ceremony, together with the names of the contractors, architect, Governor of the colony, and the Ministry of the day.*[20]

At the beginning of 1884, Garryowen was bursting at the seams with one hundred and fifty patients. Relief came in September as the first ward in the Kirkbride Complex, Ward Three for 'intermediate' male patients,[21] was opened. Kirkbride had taken four years and nine months to be born and at a cost of £250,000.[22] It could comfortably hold 766 men and women.[23] Blaxland's hospital was now split between Garryowen and its weatherboard extension, and the new buildings of the Kirkbride Complex. Work was still being completed overall, with the one hundred and fifty patients drafted in to assist. This mix of workers – patients and the tradesmen hired by Low and Kerr – did not always co-exist in harmony: in Blaxland's *Report* for the year of 1884 he noted the frustration with which the patients worked in the gardens, often having their planting trampled by the contractors.[24] By December all the patients had been transferred, at considerable trouble and stress:

> *... with very considerable labour on the part of the Attendants, and no small anxiety and trouble on the part of the Superintendent and officers, the whole of the patients have been removed from the old buildings; 61 males have been removed from* [the temporary hospital for the insane at] *Cooma, and a considerable number admitted, and during the last few days twelve females were received from Gladesville.*[25]

By the end of 1884, Callan Park was home to 270 patients: 258 men and 12 women. Still Garryowen was not finished with however: though the patients were in at Kirkbride, the kitchens there were not operational yet and those at Garryowen continued to be used to feed the men and women living and working at the hospital.

The Kirkbride Complex is a series of sandstone pavilion-style buildings built around a rectangular shape. The drainpipes are copper, and there are numerous embellishments over the walls and windows which demonstrate Barnet's attention to detail, and Manning's urgency to create in Callan Park a place of beauty. From the perspective of the front block, the left side was for men, with the engine room, stables, mortuary and carpenters' sheds, and the right side, with the laundry, for women. The place is roughly mirror-image and definitely so in terms of the wards. In the centre of the grounds is the recreation hall, and everywhere there are covered walkways and large open green spaces. There are – and were – no bars on the windows or heavy iron doors.

The front Administration block, which would have looked out over the sunken gardens, and towards the boundary on Balmain Road, is a large and beautiful beginning to the site. The gardens were the work of Mr Charles Moore, curator of the Botanical Gardens, and Mr John Sheahan, responsible for the laying out of the Crystal Palace grounds[26] and added a calm and beautiful outlook from the front building. Its stately entrance is a wonderful example of masonry, with black and white tiling at the main door. Grand though it might be, the windows and door are of a regular size: there is nothing here to intimidate or scare. It is improbable that patients would have arrived at this entrance, but rather visitors and family members. Along from the entrance hall here was an inviting reception room for patients to meet with their friends and family. Further along was the library, full of the same books donated to, and bought by, the hospital. In 1886 Blaxland petitioned for £150 for new books[27] and in 1889 Mr R. McDowall, Callan Park's Engineer, donated a complete Dickens to the library. At the edge of this front block, on the far right hand side, was Blaxland's private residence, where his children were born. This block also contained the general store and associated offices, an inquest room, various offices, and the residences of the dispenser and chief attendant, Little.

Following on around the left hand of this entrance block, beyond the dispenser's residence, were the male wards. Ward One, for convalescent patients, was the first, and created the south-east corner of the site. Ward Two, for the refractory patients, was next with its secure and enclosed airing court. Ward Three, for intermediate patients, made up the south-west corner of the site and faced back towards Garryowen. Making up part of the west side of Kirkbride, parallel to the Entrance Block, was Ward Four for newly arrived patients, and Ward Five or the Hospital Ward. Each ward was equipped with its own set of dormitories and leisure spaces. As an average, patients in New South Wales were provided with twenty-six feet of indoor space per person, almost half of what was provided in Britain.[28] It was reasoned that because Australian patients were outside a great deal more, this was roughly equal. Dormitories were generally on the top floors – of the three-storey pavilion blocks – with the lower floors used as day rooms, as the English and Scotch Boards of Lunacy preferred.[29]

Verandahs ran around the day rooms and offered shade in the airing courts. Airing courts were always attended, with the patients under observation to prevent the scaling of walls, but no other restraint was used and patients were able to walk freely around.[30] The numerous animals and pets which were regularly donated to the hospital appear to have been relatively free in the grounds of these airing courts. In 1888 Blaxland wrote that,

> *The wards are plentifully supplied with pets of all kinds. Parrots, magpies, wild-ducks, seagulls, gold-fish &c., all receive their share of attention, and I am glad to say that seldom, if ever, is any harm done to them by even the most irritable of the patients; many indeed make special favourites of them.*[31]

An image from 1903[32] shows a patient with a portable bird cage, and many of the animals presented to the patients were fit for this kind of freedom. In the early years of Callan Park, Mr Fraser donated a peacock and Blaxland's brother Francis donated a magpie. A few years later, in conjunction with a Mr A. Betts, Francis donated a long list of animals including a pair of woodland ducks and some black and mountain ducks, three wallabies and a kangaroo; Dr Cox supplied a crow and some gold and silver fish. Subsequent gifts included two pairs of black swans, a flying squirrel, another peacock and an emu.[33] When Manning witnessed a similar display during his 1868 tour, he noticed that 'at the Leicester Asylum, the aviaries for pheasants &c., in the courts, are made out of the old wire guards formerly over the windows. Thus swords have been converted into ploughshares'.[34]

The five male pavilions, besides the day rooms, each also contained a ward kitchen and store room. Attendants' rooms were also on the ground floor.[35] There were lavatories on all floors, with a bath in each. The dormitories were nicely decorated with large windows, coloured blinds, and were brightly painted.[36] They were well-lit and homely with pictures on the walls and ornaments on display. In 1884 HMS *Lark* donated two pairs of South Sea Island shells and some native weapons for the amusement of the patients.[37] Manning himself also donated a framed picture in 1888.[38]

The layout of the sleeping floors varied considerably according to the type of patient housed within. Ward One, with its convalescents, contained open dormitories with beds for twenty-eight men each. Ward Two, for violent and noisy patients, contained a variety of sleeping arrangements. There were some small associated dormitories for patients in more stable states of mind. Otherwise, there were small individual rooms reserved for violent patients, particularly ill patients, or serial escapees. These rooms were easily made secure and able to contain troublesome patients by the simple locking of the door; alternatively, for patients recovering from some seizure or fit and who required rest, these were also very useful. In the entire hospital there were 140 ordinary single rooms.[39] In addition, there were twelve panelled rooms, which were easily cleaned in the event of incontinence or other more active habits.

There were other rooms in Ward Two specifically used for the seclusion of patients in a particularly aggressive or troublesome state of mind – and these were padded. There were eight of these rooms across the male and female divisions of Callan Park: 'The padded cells are simply rooms the walls of which are upholstered with strong leather fixed upon springs, something like the partitions of first-class railway compartments, and in which it is next to impossible for a patient to do himself an injury'.[40] Manning wrote extensively on the use of such rooms as these, perhaps to dispel the myth so prominent in the public imagination of stone wall cells and screaming men, despite what might have been the case at Garryowen. He emphasised in his writing that such rooms should have windows to ensure the patient was calm and orientated. Even wire guards, he wrote, were avoided.[41] Moral Therapy preferred the *confinement* of such patients rather than the *tying up* of such men. In 1895 the definition of 'seclusion' was changed in New South Wales to align with the UK Board's understanding – that a patient in a single room with the door closed counted as one in seclusion 'whether in bed or not'. As a result, Callan Park's number of secluded patients sky-rocketed on paper, and staff were forced to adopt a method to distinguish between patients in single rooms and those 'traditionally' secluded due to their behaviour – by labelling them A and B patients.

Ward Three, for intermediate patients, contained open dormitories similar to those in Ward One, but these were smaller, with a maximum of fifteen men per room.[42] Ward Four, for the newly arrived patients, contained a mixture of individual rooms and associated dormitories. In this ward new arrivals would be assessed for approximately a month. They were monitored relatively closely, and upon diagnosis would then be transferred to Wards One, Two or Three. Ward Four was purposely situated, like the Hospital Ward (Ward Five) in the block containing the medical officers' quarters. The patients in these two wards were most likely to require urgent medical treatment and were thus located near medical help. The Hospital Ward contained two isolation rooms to quarantine patients should the need have arrived. The hospital was remarkably willing to remove patients from one ward to another based on behaviour or symptoms. Patients continually in seclusion or exhibiting troublesome tendencies were quickly transferred to Ward Two and when recovered were then removed to Ward Three or One.

The Medical Officers' Wing was the opulent centre of the west-facing wall, watching over the boat house and water edge, and was wedged between the male and female sides of the institution. In 1892, during a time of overcrowding at the hospital, it was declared that the medical officers' section of the asylum was being 'monopolized' by the medical men of Callan Park. 'The front of the building,' the New South Wales parliament was told, 'is capable of holding 200 patients'[43] and yet housed a half-dozen doctors only. In this block was the dispensary, waiting rooms, consulting rooms, and various staff spaces including apartments for the accommodation of students on placement from the University of Sydney.[44]

The five male wards were grouped around the male bath house. Aside from the normal showering and bathing facilities here were several contraptions designed to cure patients through the calming effects of water. In his 1868 book, Manning described the ideal hospital bathroom:

> *A fair-sized room, with slate or cement floor, fitted with stools for the patients to sit on, and foot-pans, supplied with water of different degrees of heat, will serve all purposes. The patients can use the foot-pans, sit on the stools and be well soaped, and finally washed by the Attendants, by means of hose of small size fixed to the water-taps. This plan of washing is used to some extent at the Sussex Asylum, the water being dashed over the patients by means of bowls; and in the new bath house at the New York City Asylum, it is proposed to fit up a room for this purpose. It is certainly more cleanly than the ordinary bath, where the same water is used for several in succession, and will take less water than it, if fresh water is used for each one.*
>
> *For treatment, ordinary baths will be necessary, but one or two will suffice in the general bath-room, instead of one to twenty or every thirty patients, which is the necessary proportion when they are used for purposes of cleanliness as well. A shower-bath is useful in certain cases, but one for each sex will be sufficient. The Turkish-bath has been found extremely useful in the treatment of various forms of insanity. Both of these should be placed in the bath house. A fixed bath will be necessary in the division for the more*

excited class of cases, since it is frequently undesirable to move them from their special section of the asylum; and one, either fixed or moveable, for use in the infirmary.[45]

Callan Park's bath house was similar to this vision, and also contained a Turkish bath or hot air bath. In such a contraption, the patient would sit in a tiled room something like a sauna, at 70°C to 90°C. The theory was that this treatment softened the skin, increased circulation and encouraged sleep. One doctor in Ireland also thought patients benefited since the 'odour of the insane' was removed by such a process.[46] Due to Callan Park's ongoing water supply issue, first noted during the fire in the top floor of Garryowen in 1881, there were issues with the Turkish bath for several years and it was not fully functioning until 1890 – six years after the patients moved into the Kirkbride complex.[47]

The mirror image to these male wards and bath house was the female division. The female side of Callan Park used the same numbering system and layout as the men. Unlike the male wards, the female wards were opened progressively as more women were admitted, with the last ward, Ward Five, being opened sometime in 1886.[48] They were decorated with the same care and attention as the men's rooms:

> *Sweetness and light may be said to be the dominant ideas throughout the institution, the former exemplified in the scrupulous cleanliness of the dormitory, the wards, and the culinary and domestic departments, the latter in the well-lighted corridors and wards and sleeping apartments, decorated with engravings and other ornaments. The courtyards are profusely adorned with flowers and shrubs, and the walls of the buildings made gay with the bright blossoms of floral climbers.*[49]

It is under the female Ward Eight that the famous Callan Park 'tunnels' or 'basements' are situated. This space, stone and rather dismal, is relatively large, and in some sections is divided into what at first sight might appear to be individual rooms. But how likely it is that these would have been used to house patients of any disposition is a hotly debated topic – given their *presumed* absolute incompatibility with the compassion of Moral Therapy. It is true that the Bethlem (or Bedlam) which Manning visited in his 1868 tour had installed basement 'cells' in 1844, but there is no evidence whatsoever that this area of Callan Park was ever used for patients in the early decades of the hospital. Visitors to Callan Park today are often unwavering believers of this space being strong evidence of the mistreatment of Victorian-era patients and are inclined to forget the details of the location of these so called 'cells' – under the wards for relatively calm women – in their quest for evidence of sadists at early Callan Park. Surely, had Manning built a secret underground ward for seriously violent or contrary patients, he would have made the site of such a place under Ward Two for violent men? It is hard to envision struggling refractory men being wrestled by attendants across the hospital all the way to – of all places – the female side of the Kirkbride Complex, past women tending the flower beds, sewing and mending, and getting all the way down a narrow staircase just for a short stint of imprisonment. Much more likely is that this cool, underground space – created by necessity since Kirkbride is built upon uneven and sloping ground – was used as a storeroom. But basements can have more than one use, of course. If George Morton was truthful in saying he was kept underground at Garryowen, then perhaps the Kirkbride 'basements' *were* used for such purposes. It is interesting to note that 'dark rooms' were not seen as in opposition to Moral Therapy,[50] so long as patients were not mechanically restrained while there. They were in fact used fairly frequently throughout the Commonwealth, as places were patients would lack stimulation and find peace, calmness and – most often – sleep. If we consider this space as a last resort method of treatment, where patients could be cool and calm, then perhaps it was not so very cruel a place – despite the popular images of abuse it conjures up even today. Its use as a storeroom is, however, more persuasive.

The expected industry of each sex at Callan Park was made clear by the situation of various sheds and studios in the Kirkbride Complex. On the female side was the magnificent laundry and sewing room; on the men's side were the carpenter's and painter's shops, the engine room and stables.

The laundry was a large room with various ante rooms. The main area contained two large revolving washing machines and three 'hydro-extractors'. There were four large boiling vats for the disinfecting of clothes and linen, and seventeen brick and cement washing troughs – with both hot and cold water – along with two wringers. Beyond this room was the drying room which contained seventeen Bradford's patent drying horses. The system was quite complex:

> *Each horse travels along a pair of rails, and is drawn out to have clothes placed upon it for drying, when it is pushed back into its place, the outer end forming an iron door when the airer is in position. This keeps the hot air in, as, when all the airers are in their place that part occupied by the clothes is like an immense oven, the interior of which is heated by the steam pipes, and so the clothes can be regularly and well dried, independent altogether of the state of the atmosphere. A steel coil, heated by the passage of steam through the pipes, is used for drying horse hair, or mattresses if need be.*[51]

In addition, there was a separate washing room for the staff linen. This also appears to have been worked by patients.

The steam upon which the laundry and bath house relied was generated by the engine room on the male side of the complex. The engine was connected to three very large boilers and a Tangye duplex pump which supplied the entire site with hot water.[52] This was connected to the large water tanks under the site, filled via the pipes attached to the verandahs. The tanks held over 1,880,000 gallons[53] and were connected to the magnificent clock tower in the centre of the site. This water tower, which never received its clock faces, contains a visible copper ball which rises and falls according to the quantity of water in the underground tanks. Aside from bathing and washing, this water was also essential in the event of a fire. In 1885 Mr Bear, the superintendent of the Metropolitan Fire Brigades, audited Callan Park and concluded, due to the inability of fire crews to quickly reach the site, that the hospital needed to be self-sufficient in fire-fighting.[54] Blaxland regarded his staff as very fine in their attention to this: once a fortnight Mr Bear sent an instructor to teach the attendants at Callan Park how to manage a fire and 'brought the attendants up to a very creditable standard of efficiency'.[55]

Across from the engine room and along from the stables, was the Mortuary, near the gates leading out of the asylum beside male Ward One. It was here where post-mortems were carried out after the deaths of patients, and where corpses were collected to be taken to the wide number of cemeteries used by Callan Park. Some space in the nearby stables was to house the hearse which would be used in the event of a patient's death. There is no evidence to suggest that patients were ever buried on site as they had been at the pre-Manning Gladesville. Most patients were buried in local cemeteries including Balmain Cemetery and Rookwood, in plots which are still recorded and locatable today. Only the burial places of some very few patients, and usually Chinese or African men with no family and difficult names, have been lost to history.

In the centre of the Kirkbride Complex were the dining and recreation rooms. The recreation hall was a commodious room set with a stage at one end, before an ornate stained-glass window which is still visible today. In 1895 the stage was described as having been embellished with an 'astrological canopy' and 'emblazoned' with the hospital's patriotic and not unique motto, *Domine salvum fac reginam*,[56] 'Lord, make the Queen safe'. Here events were often held – plays and musical amusements on the stage, and the polished floor was often used for dances, including fancy dress parties with the patients from other similar institutions. In 1885 Blaxland initiated a regular dance at Callan Park for the patients now that he had the space, held once a month[57] and from 1887, balls were held each year. In 1888 the event made the newspaper, described as 'a most successful and enjoyable affair'. The ball was 'given by the nurses and attendants' of Callan Park, and, aside from their equals at Gladesville and Parramatta being invited, forty of the 'more advanced patients also participated in the evening's enjoyment' which lasted until one o'clock in the morning. The ballroom was 'most artistically decorated with flags of all nations' and attendants Carter and Dempsy oversaw the event as MCs.[58] In 1886 Blaxland congratulated his staff for taking the time to rehearse and perform a farce for the patients in the recreation hall[59] and in 1887 a fireworks display was put on for all of Callan Park's residents.[60]

On Sundays the recreation hall doubled as a chapel, and it is reasonable to assume the harmonium which caused so much excitement at Garryowen in its early days found a new home there. Manning was rather concerned at this double use of the recreation hall, writing in 1868:

> [It is] *a matter of debate whether the room appropriated for dancing and amusement should be used as a chapel also, or whether a room should be specially set apart for religious service only; and, if set apart, whether it should be in the main building or detached.*[61]

In consultation with Barnet, he seems to have quietened the debate in his mind and settled for a convertible, multi-purpose room.

The dining rooms, on either side of the recreation hall, catered separately for both men and women and was where the majority of patients went for their meals. Those patients of a violent or unpredictable nature, in either the male or female sides of the asylum, ate their meals in their own wards.[62] Of course, in massing such disparate patients together for meals in the halls, some issues occurred. In 1891 Blaxland noted in his *Annual Report* that contraband in one ward not being the same in another, often banned items could be passed during such meetings.[63] Blaxland was not specific about the kind of items, but it is possible he referred to articles of clothing, or even tools. It is likely that patients would have assisted in the serving of meals and the clearing of plates at the end, particularly as the hospital grew in size. Attendants would have been on hand to count cutlery back into the kitchen to ensure no knives made their way into the wrong hands. Shutters which ran down one side of both the male and female dining areas allowed the recreation hall to expand to a much larger space.[64]

Next door, within a small distance to this small arrangement of rooms, was the kitchen, another venue for patients to assist and work. The kitchen was well-equipped with three large Cornish steel boilers[65] connected to the steam engine a little way off in the male division. The kitchen itself was thirty-nine feet by twenty feet. It contained one seven-foot cooking range, two tea boilers, three large and four small 'soup boilers', a large 'steam cutting up table', a scullery and one range 'consisting of three potato steamers, one cabbage boiler, two fat and bone boilers, two dough troughs and one baker's oven'.[66] The food, much of it grown on site, was wholesome. Manning was very keen that the food be varied and interesting and fresh: something to look forward to each day.[67]

Other than these main blocks were the accessory buildings, including a bakehouse, flour store, dining rooms for attendants and nurses (manned by well-behaved patients), store-rooms for clothing and provisions (again, run by patients), carpenters', painters', tailors', and shoe-makers' shops; a shed for bricklayers, and sewing rooms.[68] These were all connected by asphalted verandahs – in total, 1.25 miles of undercover access[69] – and by 1888, reliable telephonic connection and a working bell-system[70] which replaced the much slower dispatch of messengers in times needing of medical assistance or in calling some patient to meet his or her visitors.

Thus stood the new Kirkbride Complex of Callan Park, surrounded by acres of good farmland. Up near Balmain Road still stood the cricket paddock which had been initiated by Blaxland when the asylum had worked from Garryowen. Now, a tennis court was added[71] and the cricket pitch bounded by a nine-foot fence to allow the patients privacy from the people walking past the pitch, and who were liable to call out 'irritating remarks which the patients naturally resented'[72]. At the same time, a pavilion – designed by an ex-patient[73] – was erected with dressing rooms and seats for spectators. Down at the water, towards Iron Cove, Blaxland for many years continued to utilize the Department's steam-launch as 'one form of recreation which was greatly enjoyed, especially by the women'.[74] He allowed tours of the harbour, and found it was also a convenient and amusing method of transport to picnics and other events. In 1887, the boat was given over to the 'services of a gentleman engaged in exploring New Guinea' and Callan Park's patients were thus deprived. But by 1889 a new boat, *Mabel,* had been offered and was seen as a valuable control on the female patients in particular, who Blaxland described in his *Annual Report*: 'many of the turbulent [female patients] ... will frequently exercise considerable self-control for a long period in order to get an 'outing' [on *Mabel*]'.[75] In addition, patients continued to amuse themselves with quoits, rounders and skittles.[76] The farming areas also received an added boost with the building in 1889 of a proper farm house in which the resident farm attendant might live.[77] The unusual layout of this building, with several small rooms, indicates its possible use as a place of patient accommodation. One of Manning's pioneering ideas – that convalescent patients almost ready to be discharged be thus distributed away from the Kirkbride buildings – was to have patients living in the farm house and the gate house on Balmain Road.[78] The construction of this farm building however was originally in response to a large amount of stealing from the vegetable garden and also farm sheds, including bran and bones.[79]

Garryowen or the 'Old House' as it came to be termed, was not forsaken in this new era, but rather reincorporated into the new hospital. In his original survey of New South Wales and its care for the mentally ill in the 1860s, Manning had observed in New South Wales the lack of both private institutions for the insane, and provisions in state institutions for the better off or higher class of patients. He wrote in 1868, 'At present there is no provision in any asylum for patients of a superior class ... In the design of a new public asylum, especial attention should be paid to this point, and an express reservation made for the reception of such patients'.[80] Manning had a particular dislike of the use of cottages to treat the majority of patients. He complained that they were more expensive to build, staff and supervise[81] – particularly in terms of efficiency in medical care – and that as a result, to use cottages for the common patient was unwise and possibly dangerous. For convalescents of the 'superior class' however, used to cosy and cultured surroundings, they were ideal as they created a comfortable and familiar-type home.[82] To provide this 'higher level' of care in the state's asylums was an attempt to change the public perception of such institutions. There was no law in New South Wales requiring the confinement of anyone showing symptoms of insanity, and as a result 'better class' men and women who were insane were likely to be cared for on an individual basis or through private practice. It meant that men and women confined in *asylums* were usually of a poorer class, or those without family support. In the public opinion, this created a stronger than ever link between criminality, poverty and insanity.[83] Welcoming upper-class patients to the state's asylums was an attempt to break this prevailing preconception.

1882 brought a dramatic change in Legard's fortune. Continuing to call Ward Two at Garryowen home, and as the Kirkbride Complex came to life just down the hill, he was still collecting rubbish and working a little in the grounds. There were small scuffles with other Ward Two patients: at one point Samuel Payne blackened his eye and Legard, now seventy years old, retaliated this time with verbal abuse rather than violence. But over on the other side of the world, in England, Legard's two remaining sisters were dying. By December they were both dead. No doubt to the surprise of even himself, Legard and his brother William Barnabas, whose wife coincidently was a lunatic at the infamous Bedlam Asylum, were the two surviving children of their household, and now they came into their money. Immediately the master-in-lunacy began charging Legard's account for his care in the state asylum system out of his mother's – albeit stingy – annuity. Legard paid the full rate at Callan Park: £65 per year (paid in quarterly instalments of £16, 5s) and was one of the few patients in a position to do so. He was termed a 'Master's Pay Patient' and later a 'Master's Patient', meaning that the master-in-lunacy had full control over his finances, due to the lack of friends or relatives who might be called on in a similar instance to forward the payments for his care. Manning had unwittingly delivered to Callan Park, in the first batch of forty-four patients, exactly the type of patient he wished to increase in the state system. Legard's culture and education was exactly what Manning was hoping to cater for in the cottages he had designed on the fringe of Callan Park's Kirkbride complex.

There is no doubt that Legard's name would have been first on the list of patients transferred to the ward specially designed for paying patients – for men, a renovated Garryowen House. But the old mansion was not ready for patients until 1888 – and neither was Legard, who continued to be housed in

Ward Two even in the Kirkbride Complex when it opened. He was 'in fair bodily health' but dirty, angry, abusive. One comment, that he would 'always be 'on medicine', what, does not matter', demonstrates the consistency of his hypochondriacal tendencies and obsessive behaviour. In March 1884 it was decided that he was 'too mischievous to be kept at work' and he was often secluded for excess noise and excitement. In 1885 he had his nose broken by another patient, he was erratic in speech and 'deficient in power of attention'. But finally in 1888 when Garryowen was opened as a retreat for paying patients, Legard escaped Kirkbride's Ward Two and found quiet and tranquillity within the walls of the old mansion.

Living in Garryowen, removed from the noise and excitement of the Kirkbride Complex, would have been like living in a normal cottage in the outside world. Legard would have found comfort in this – harking back to his childhood and early career in Ganton, and in Brighton Park. The place had originally been a home, the residence of Brenan and Gordon, and now it was again. The standard of living here was higher than over at Kirkbride, and pains were taken to decorate the cottage in the style of a normal home. The records for Legard covering the period of 1887 to 1890 are very brief and are likely a result of his calm time in the old mansion away from the stresses and triggers of Kirkbride. Legard would have spent his time working on his arithmetic and using the libraries of Callan Park.

Garryowen was the ideal site to accommodate these socially 'better' patients in New South Wales' first semi-private male ward. The Old Mansion's grandeur and stateliness recommended it as a perfect location for Manning's experiment and needed only a small extension to the west, completed in 1885, to make it worthwhile. Close enough to the Kirkbride Complex for medical help, but also secluded enough to provide a clear spatial 'difference' to its patients, Garryowen became home to the state's first full-paying patients. Garryowen appears to have been self-sufficient, rather than dependant on Kirkbride, as its old laundry was converted to a store and larder.[84] A little along the road behind the Medical Officer's Wing of Kirkbride was built the female equivalent. Both were opened in 1888[85] and were a source of great contentment for the patients thus installed: 'The patients residing in these buildings have special accommodation. Their meals and their surroundings are more in consonance with their usual manner of living before entering the hospital, and they evidently appreciate what is done for their comfort'. In 1889, upon an inspection of both, Manning reported with some pride:

> *The detached buildings set apart for paying patients in the male division are working satisfactorily. The rooms are cheerful and are well furnished, the dietary scale is a liberal one, and the comfort of the patients well attended to. The gardens are well kept, and attending to the flower-beds affords agreeable occupation to some of the patients. The rooms are not yet fully occupied, but are filling up gradually.*[86]

These patients paid handsomely for the privilege of this accommodation. Three-quarters of the minimum wage at the time,[87] or £5 18s per month, bought a place in one of these private wards. Callan Park did not make a significant profit from even these patients however: in 1887 it was estimated that the cost of keeping each patient was between £60 and £70 per year,[88] which was approximately the maximum that these patients were charged. Patients who could contribute to their upkeep were obliged to do so and made payment via the master-in-lunacy. £3 8s was the cost of a place in an ordinary ward in the Kirkbride Complex if one was able to pay it.[89] The ledgers kept by the master-in-lunacy reveal a wide range of payments being made by the friends and family of patients, or the patients themselves if they had no next of kin (and were called Master's Pay Patients like Legard). Sums ranging from 12s to £5 per month were recorded, along with the occasional alteration in payments, usually a reduction, during leaner times.

The question of 'better class' patients in both private and state-run asylums was a topical issue at the time. By 1888, there were 130 state patients being cared for at the private Cook's River Asylum, at great cost to the government. As in the state institutions, some of these contributed to the cost of their treatment. Run then by Dr Arthur Vause, Bayview was not now known for its high level of care. In 1880 the antiquated appliances and run-down nature of the site had been noted.[90] As a result, in 1894, a Royal Commission into the 'Conduct and Management of the Licensed House for the Insane at Cook's River' was opened and many patients were removed in response. One patient, unnamed in the *New South Wales Legislative Assembly* papers,[91] who was paying somewhere between £200 and £300 per year for residence there, was removed first to Callan Park, provoking much scandal in the New South Wales parliament. The anger stemmed from the privilege this man enjoyed at the expense of other less wealthy patients. One member of parliament complained, 'I say, that the Government and their officers were failing in their duty in not at once removing the fifty patients when they removed the one gentleman to Callan Park.' He continued, somewhat sarcastically, 'It would naturally be expected that an inmate for whom £200 or £300 a year was paid would be treated in a far better manner than ordinary Government patients.' He went on to add,

> *If it was right and proper for the Government official to remove the one unfortunate, who is supposed to be well looked after by the payment on the part of his friends of £200 or £300 a year, if it was right to remove him because of ill-treatment, then God help the poor unfortunate fifty who have not any friends to look after them; and I say that this House and the Government ought now, with this knowledge before them, to immediately remove these patients, a clear case having been made out of ill-treatment in the case of one patient. There is too much danger in allowing these poor unfortunates to remain in this establishment any longer.*[92]

In 1890, it was noted that those at Garryowen were not perhaps progressing as had been hoped, and elements of Moral Therapy began to break down within the walls of the privileged house:

> *The cottages for paying and better class male patients have been fully occupied, and have worked satisfactorily, being comfortable and homelike. Some difficulty, however, is experienced in inducing*

the patients to occupy themselves usefully, as they do not appear to realize the beneficial effects of work, and some consider that as they are paying full rates for maintenance, they should not be asked to occupy themselves. One of the buildings – the old mansion – is very old, and in constant need of minor repairs. A large part of the flooring on the ground floor will soon have to be renewed, and, owing to damp walls, the papering does not last as long as it should.[93]

In 1891, a year after his brother William Barnabas died, Legard dropped off the master-in-lunacy's ledger of paying patients. This coincided with an increase in notes in his file. It is likely that this indicated a removal from Garryowen due to his advanced age. Legard, the youngest child of Cecilia and William Legard, was seventy-nine now, and had out-lived all of his brothers and sisters. He was likely transferred to Ward Five, the Hospital Ward, at Kirkbride. His advanced age protected him from the mass transfer of patients from the over-crowded Callan Park in the early 1890s to other of the state's asylums.

Next door to Garryowen in the weatherboard buildings originally meant as a temporary measure to house the refractory patients in the late 1870s were the 'more demented and hopeless [chronic] patients'.[94] Blaxland's irritation concerning these patients is well-recorded: he regarded many of these men as having been wrongly brought to Callan Park, and better-suited to care in a poorhouse rather than a hospital for the insane. In 1887 there was an influx of such men from the Coast Hospital at Little Bay. Blaxland, while acknowledging their mental 'deficiency' noted that they were wrongly allowed admittance by the department since their bodily ailments could have been treated elsewhere.[95]

And so Callan Park was made. Kirkbride was the centre of the hospital now, and Garryowen home to the superior paying patients of the institution. The farm was extensive, the gardens magnificent – and even more so with the donation of a handsome cast iron bench from Messrs Hyde and Sons in 1884[96] – and the cricket paddock in constant use. Manning's dream was realised with Blaxland at the helm. New South Wales' institutions were the envy of the country and Commonwealth in terms of design and intentions. But sandstone bricks and good intentions are not necessarily indicators of the reality of any place. Manning's institution was indeed beautiful but what of the staff which carried out his laws and procedures? The quality of life for Callan Park's residents was in their hands. It was the attendants who made the place what it was. Were they rough punishers of the madmen under their control, as Reade and Perceval would have us believe persisted throughout the world? Or were Manning's employees made in his own image – benevolent humane carers of the insane?

4

ATTENDANTS AND THE ROUTINE

By the late 1890s Callan Park was joined by several other institutions opened under Manning's watch.

In 1888 a branch establishment of Parramatta was opened at Rydalmere but was not called the Rydalmere Hospital for the Insane until 1892. This asylum was housed in the buildings formerly known as the Protestant Orphan School and relieved the over-crowding at all the major metropolitan institutions. The first of Manning's 'up country' asylums was also built in Goulburn. Called Kenmore, and opened in 1894, this hospital allowed patients from rural backgrounds to be cared for closer to friends and family.

Manning's impressive system of six major hospitals – Callan Park, Gladesville, Parramatta and Rydalmere in Sydney, and Kenmore and Newcastle thus removed – worked together to manage the ever-increasing number of insane in the colony. Just before the turn of the century, Rydalmere and Morisset (opened in 1906) and Kenmore were the major centres used in the housing of chronic patients and came to have a custodial rather than medical emphasis.[1] Callan Park and Gladesville became the hospitals for the reception of acute patients and were therefore hubs of medical training and evolution. As a result, the ledgers for these institutions demonstrate a high turnover of patients – ending quickly in either discharge or transfer to an institution dealing in long term care. Parramatta, still with its criminal division, worked both sides of the equation, with both chronic and acute patients. Conversely, Newcastle continued with its emphasis on children, opening a school in 1908, and on the care of 'idiots'. The private asylum at Cook's River continued and was joined in 1893 by a second private, and very small, institution in Ryde, Mount St Margaret. In 1887 an unlicensed private house in Picton, containing two lunatics, had charges brought against it.[2] Other than this, the landscape of New South Wales remained safely in the hands of state-run insane hospitals.

Numbers of staff and their wages were largely consistent throughout these institutions. Under the medical superintendent was a strict hierarchy of staff – with university-educated medical men at the top, attendants and nurses as carers with a middling place in the order of things, and a veritable army of artisans, workmen and servants at the bottom.

Blaxland as medical superintendent was entirely responsible for running Callan Park. By the 1890s he had come to earn £700 a year[3] for the privilege of hiring and sacking staff, liaising with the Inspector General, adhering to the relevant Lunacy Laws and Acts and sustaining the general health and well-being of both staff and patients. Medical superintendents necessarily lived onsite and were on call 24/7. Both Blaxland and Scholes were involved in urgent medical assistance (such as instances of choking) and planned surgery. Blaxland's identification with both Callan Park and Gladesville – in their cricketing teams and winning horticultural prizes on the hospitals' behalf – demonstrates the residential nature of the role.

The assistant superintendent at Callan Park in the early days before 1900 was the clerk Arthur Whitling. Whitling's job was to ensure the bureaucracy of Callan Park ran smoothly. Death certificates were signed by him, and correspondence from the Department of Lunacy was managed in his office. From 1885 Whitling was assisted by a junior clerk, Charles H. Richardson, who earned a little over half the salary of Whitling, at £170 per annum.

Under these men in the institution's hierarchy were the medical officers, housed in their grand wing of the Kirkbride Complex, and led by an assistant medical officer to the superintendent. The first assistant medical officer at Callan Park was Dr David Grant in 1885, who was quickly replaced by the long-employed Dr George Edward Miles in 1886, due to ill health. It was part of the assistant medical officer's role to act as superintendent when required by the absence of Blaxland. The medical officers were required to hold a diploma in surgery and were to be in the wards daily, preparing medicines with the assistance of the dispenser John T. Floyd, assessing patients and, where needed, taking upon themselves the duties of assistant medical officer should he be unavailable or incapacitated.[4] From all accounts, Manning experienced some difficulty in filling these positions due to the limited salary the government could offer[5] compared to other medical posts in the colony.

The constant presence in the wards was that of the attendants. The twenty-one junior attendants and, initially, a team of twelve senior attendants of Callan Park in 1885, were managed by chief attendant William Little, one of the pallbearers at Manning's funeral[6] and who rose to the station of chief attendant in the Lunacy Department.[7] Senior attendants were paid between £90 and £102 per year and junior attendants between £72 and £84. This changed within the decade, and by 1896, further stratification in attendants had been created: now Little managed a team of eight 'attendants in charge of wards' – all names which occurred frequently in the medical notes of patients and many of whom had been at Callan Park as a branch establishment: Bulfin, Thomas Skerritt (whose brother Harry worked as an attendant at Gladesville Hospital)[8], Carter, Hain, Cashman, Dempsey, Love and Dwyer and paid £130 per annum – who managed twelve senior attendants (£125 per year) and multiple juniors (at £108).[9] Of the vast numbers of attendants, some had special duties. By 1896 there was an outdoor attendant, a store attendant, a hall attendant and a farm attendant, who supervised patients while working in locations beyond that of the wards.

Callan Park also employed numerous nurses in its Hospital Wards on either side of the medical officers' quarters. In 1885, when the Kirkbride Complex was only new, there were four senior nurses (at £60 to £50 per year) and eight junior nurses (£40 to 46) answerable to the matron, Marian A. Fairbairn (£140 per year). One of these nurses in 1885 was appointed to one of the male wards as an experiment in Victorian-era healthcare. Manning, in reporting on this novel idea, wrote:

> *Among the additions to the staff Dr Blaxland, with my full concurrence, appointed a nurse to one of the male wards. The result*

has been most encouraging, the sick have been better nursed and looked after, the patients in the ward have behaved better, and it is decidedly a matter for consideration whether female nurses may not be more largely employed in the male wards if suitable persons can be found to undertake duties.[10]

The following year, Blaxland joined in with further praise: 'It has worked very satisfactorily; bed sores are of less frequency, better attention is paid to such as are physically ailing, and more tidiness and order prevail'.[11]

Of these men and women at Callan Park a select few were hired as night attendants and nurses, and were an extended part of the night 'team' who ensured gates and doors were locked and the hospital secure once the sun went down. In 1886,[12] there were four night attendants: two for the general wards, one specifically for Ward Two and one for the detached buildings. The detached buildings included Garryowen and the female cottages, the weatherboard additions for chronic convalescents and those in the farmhouse and gatekeeper's cottage. There were two night nurses for the general wards and one for Ward Two.[13] These staff members were required to complete regular examinations of the dormitories and single rooms, partly to prevent escape but also check on the health of patients. Observations were also recorded in the *Night Attendants' Book*s which have been lost to history.

In addition to this large staff were the artisans and servants of Callan Park. By 1896 Callan Park employed a needlewoman, a housemaid, two gatekeepers, five cooks, four laundresses, two engine drivers, three artisans and a gardener. The gardener was Samuel Cheetham, resident since Callan Park's inception in 1876. Cheetham, as overseer of Callan Park's increasingly elaborate gardens and farms, acquired a small degree of fame in his role, making the newspaper several times in the 1890s. In 1891 the Technical College agricultural students visited Cheetham's gardens to 'study the very excellent system of vegetable gardening allowed there' and the superior piggeries 'being among the best of their kind in the colonies'.[14] In 1898 students from Granville Technical School and Sydney College visited the vegetable gardens again 'for a practical lesson on vegetable sowing' by

Cheetham, 'a former student of the classes'.[15] In the same year, Cheetham's name was used dozens of times to advertise the quality of a particular brand of cabbage seed:

> *Shepherd's short stem cabbage. Extraordinary yield. Messrs. P.L. C. Shepherd and Son, the well-known Seedmen, of 202, Pitt-Street, Sydney, have received the following letter from Mr. T. Cheetham, of Callan Park: – 'The seed of Shepherd's short stem cabbage, supplied by you, has given the following wonderful results: – From a bed of 152 × 80 feet I cut 3 tons 7 ewt. (13 tons per acre), and one head weighted 40lb.' P.L.C. Shepherd and Son send their Catalogue free to all applicants.*[16]

The positions of Chaplain – both Church of England and Roman Catholic – were still filled, though incredulously to some: one New South Wales member of parliament wondered aloud in 1884: 'Why be at the expense of providing Church of England and Roman Catholic chaplains to preach the gospel to poor creatures who did not know their right hand from the left. Was it not like whistling a jig to a milestone? He did not want to see public money spent unnecessarily'.[17] In 1892, in an effort to curb Callan Park's expenses, the New South Wales parliament debated the benefit of religion at the hospital. One member commented,

> *I should like to know what the duties of the chaplains are? If they are supposed to preach to the lunatics, I think the best we can do is to strike out the allowance. It is very little comfort to a lunatic to have to sit and listen to some sermons ... To preach sermons to lunatics is a piece of lunacy in itself, and the practice ought to be put a stop to. The poor unfortunates have quite enough to put up with without that infliction.*[18]

But it was the attendants who dealt with patients each day, all day, and it was therefore these men whose work is most visible in the records of

Callan Park. Their successes and failures are all laid out, often in detail, in the *Medical Case Books* and *Journals* of the patients with whom they interacted. The records paint a broad picture of caring individuals who knew the patients well, but who were sometimes put upon by long hours and the stress of managing grown men who were often unpredictable, sly and mischievous. Occasionally, these attendants were men who did not know themselves well enough to realise they would not cope with their work until they were in situations they knew not how to deal with; some were brutal and managed to equate the role of attendant with that of zoo keeper. Attention to detail, a healthy cynicism and a respect for those in one's care were paramount in any attendant; physical strength, mental resilience in times of stress and a cool head were also pre-requisites. These men were not brutes; sometimes perhaps a little rash in certain circumstances, but rarely sadists. Somewhat pleasingly, Manning himself understood the weight of being an attendant. In 1868 he wrote,

> *A very little consideration of what asylum life is, – its constant worry and irritation, – the vexing influence of constant association with crooked people and crooked actions, – are felt often too severely by the asylum physicians, who are only a part of the day with the patients. The attendant has the insane always with him; and if he is to retain that health, that evenness of temper, that mental and bodily spring, that combined firmness and suavity of manner, which are necessary to make him an effective and useful servant, he must escape occasionally from the asylum walls and from the depressing influences of asylum life, and lose all thought of his work, by associating with the sane, either in the quiet of home life, or – what is and always, must be attractive to the young, and to the majority of asylum servants – the minor excitements of town life.*[19]

But allowing the attendants to 'escape occasionally' sometimes ended badly. In late 1885 and early 1886, two Callan Park attendants died during a typhoid outbreak at the hospital.[20] Robert Emerson and Michael O'Neill, the latter having only been at the park for two months prior to his death, were both unmarried and reported to have caught the disease off one of the carers of the first typhoid patient. Five members of staff were sick with the disease, but no patients were struck down. The staff were isolated at the time in one of the empty female wards as yet unopened and were treated by one of the nurses from the Hospital Wards. Manning and Blaxland, concerned at the outbreak but calmed by the lack of its spread to the patients – indicating a source outside the boundary of the asylum – investigated. Manning was described at the time as being 'somewhat affected by the circumstance'[21] and Dr Ashburton Thompson, the medical officer of the government and the president of the Board of Health, was brought in to divine the source. The source was found to be the milk from the dairy at the Helsarmel Estate at Leichardt. In the district, out of 123 houses supplied by the dairy, twenty-eight houses were infected. There was another typhoid outbreak in 1889, with a medical officer's wife, two nurses and one junior medical officer infected; none died.[22] But again in 1891 – this time the result of a severe epidemic of influenza which inundated Gladesville, Parramatta and Callan Park with a total of 736 cases (310 at Callan Park) – one attendant died.[23]

In the 1890s the work of attendants was much discussed in parliament. The general consensus was that the attendants were over-worked and burdened with excessive responsibility, increasing their likelihood of burn-out or suddenly snapping and hurting a patient. In 1892 one member of the New South Wales parliament complained, 'I paid a visit to the institution [Callan Park] the other day, and in passing through the wards I found that one attendant had to look after thirty, forty, fifty very dangerous cases in an open ward'.[24] Exactly which ward this might have been is a mystery: none of the spaces where 'dangerous' patients were held contained such large numbers, and wards were not staffed by individuals but teams of attendants. But our hyperbolic minister went on with some truth:

> *On average, attendants work for twelve and thirteen hours a day, and that they receive from £66 to £108 a year, according to their*

length of service. Of course, they get board and lodging. Considering the arduous nature of their duties, and that they continually hold their lives in their hands, the number of attendants is not sufficient, and their hours of work are far too long.[25]

These allegations – importantly criticising both the wellbeing of the staff along with the subsequent quality of the treatment of the patients – and concerns were easily countered by Manning, who clarified: 'The average number of hours on duty is eleven, and although a certain number must necessarily be on duty on Sundays, every one receives leave for fifty-two days in each year to make up for this.' He added, somewhat pointedly, 'All employed are fully aware, when engaged, of the rate of remuneration and the hours they are expected to be on duty'.[26] But the minsters had a point: 'their work is of a very arduous nature; they have to be ever on the watch, because, by the slightest mistake or absence from duty, some serious fatality might occur'.[27] Dozens of attendants *were* caring for over 700 patients. It was again pointed out: 'these men are not paid like ordinary labouring men: they are paid £8 a month ... with board, lodging and washing, and they are allowed three days in every month as a holiday'.[28]

The attendants were responsible for the daily running of the hospital and began with the morning wakeup. In the summer patients were roused from bed at 6am, and 6.30am in the winter.[29] The handover by night attendants would be done, and any events during the night – escapes, any medical events, the application of any kind of restraint – would be detailed to the attendant in charge. Staff would assist with dressing, and in some wards distribute clothing to patients. Patients would make their own beds; they would be supervised in this by the attendants and most probably the patients called 'wardsmen' who were both keen and able to assist. Breakfast was served and consisted of bread and tea. Depending on the type of patients under the care of an attendant, meals could include violence between the inmates. Violence during meals normally consisted of pushing or clapping one's attacker over the head with a tea mug, and usually as the result of some attempted theft of food. While not normally serious it still meant attendants had to be vigilant and be ready to break up any fights – and they did. At the end of the meal cutlery would be counted back into the ward's store room. The rooms would then be cleaned and patients either let out into their ward's airing court to care for the various pets or play games such as quoits – under supervision to ensure no scaling of walls or roofs – or taken to work in the grounds.

Supervising working parties was a primary role of many attendants. Attendants would pick up patients from their wards, count them out and ensure the same number was deposited back a few hours later. In the summer months it may be assumed that working parties set out early to avoid the hot afternoons. The men in these working groups worked all over the grounds, building fences, planting gardens, maintaining the grounds, painting and building. The reward for such service was extra food: half a pint of beer with bread and cheese for lunch in addition to their normal meal; lime juice could be substituted for the beer in the case of the non-drinkers, or those were required to abstain as part of their treatment. Women who worked – in the laundry or workroom, sewing – received the same bread and cheese, along with coffee at lunch and tea in the afternoon.[30] For some, the reward was even greater: working parties, where patients vastly outnumbered the one or two attendants supervising, were ideal opportunities for escape, particularly when the group was working near the far reaches of the park, near the road.

Escapees – from working parties, wards, anywhere – were generally tracked by the attendants, and only occasionally with the help of police. It was the attendants who were obliged to chase these sly men and women who suddenly vaulted from their room or garden bed. Often the attendant in charge of a working party or ward caught the patient before they had gotten too far: stories of patients being discovered hanging out of windows, mid-way through their daring vanishing act, or sauntering towards the main gate on Balmain Road only to be chased down within the hour, were common. But patients who really did go missing would often find themselves under a week-long surveillance by attendants outside their place of refuge or be cornered at some far away suburb and brought back. Arthur Brown,[31] a thirty-year old sailor suffering from a delusional form of melancholia caused supposedly by masturbation, acts as a prime example of such a process. In April 1885

Brown, who had previously been cared for privately and had only been at Callan Park for a short time, escaped from Ward One. The tailor, with whom he had been working, did not officially hand Brown over to the ward attendant, and Brown became aware that he was not supervised. He decided to make the most of this and climb a verandah post close to the boundary wall and escape. It took until the next day for the two attendants – who were both fined for their incompetence – to retake Brown. Patrick Daly, one of the attendants, 'was at once sent in pursuit' with Redfern police officer McColl, and discovered Brown the next day at his sister's house in Bullanaming Street.

As such, attendants formed the front line of the Callan Park staff and were thus often in the firing line. Attendants were frequently outlets for violent patients in particularly aggressive moods or inmates who were keen to cause trouble; in such interactions, it was often difficult for attendants to successfully gauge the amount of force necessary to both protect themselves and compel the patients in their charge to follow instructions. In 1882 attendant Lowett[32] was reprimanded for struggling with a patient rather than calling for assistance. In this case, Blaxland was a direct witness and watched as the patient Houlahan, on his way to a medical inspection, kicked Lowett and sought to hit him in the face. Blaxland described Lowett as nevertheless despite his injuries 'closing' with Houlahan and throwing him, where his forehead and mouth were injured and began to bleed. One wonders in this instance how Lowett might have called for help in such a short amount of time, particularly if he feared a continuation of the attack already begun. Why Blaxland merely watched on is also of interest even though he knew Houlahan to be 'extremely self-willed and obstinate'. But what is important to take from this instance is that Blaxland would not stand for violence to his patients; they had to be handled correctly to ensure no injury to either patient or staff. Blaxland sought to teach his staff not to seek an eye for an eye but remember that their insane charges often knew not what they did.[33]

Indeed, if anything, staff were at more risk of injury than the patients. Staff were regularly attacked with mugs and fists, and this often ended in a stint in seclusion for their assailant. In 1894 Thomas King made a sudden and homicidal attack on the farm attendant, Perryman:

> *King was working in the pig sty with a long-handled shovel and Perryman was passing along the road beside and had past* [sic] *and turned his back on King when he received a blow on the head from the shovel which knocked him down; on rising he saw King rushing towards him thro*[ugh] *the gate preparing to renew the attack when he was intercepted by another patient. Perryman received a severe but not serous scalp wound about 2 inches in length ... King was been here since January 1887 and has worked most of the time with the same attendant – invariably quiet and industrious and trustworthy and had never shown any inclination of homicidal tendencies, after the assault appeared quite unconcerned and on being asked why he committed it said 'I was told to kill Perryman yesterday and ought to have done so'.*[34]

Even attacks on Blaxland were not unheard of: Dan Cunningham was regularly placed in seclusion during the medical superintendent's medical visits due to 'his dislike of the Med[ical] Sup[erin]t[endant] at whom he has twice struck'.[35] But not all injuries were the result of malicious intentions: accidents were also common. Attendant Sherack in 1883 was tripped by a patient, Duffy, who was reluctant to attend dinner. In his notes, Blaxland recorded Duffy's injury – a small abrasion on the forehead – but not his staff's.[36]

Attendants were also responsible for the application and monitoring of any mechanical restraints decided as proper for patients. Mechanical restraints were reserved as a last resort, and only used on the most dangerous patients, to protect themselves, other patients and staff. The administration of any of these methods of restraint would have been a difficult and unenviable task, and patients who were thus restrained and had to be fed by hand were managed by attendants. Some patients, like Winders who attempted to hang himself one night in January 1886, had to be monitored regularly. Winders was confined to a camisole during the day, and muffs at night for two months until his suicidal thoughts had passed. This would most likely have been a daily struggle for the attendants caring for Winders.[37] Such patients had to be regularly checked on: it was possible to struggle out of a camisole, as evidenced by Charles Frederick Morely in 1887, a twenty-nine-year-old who used his newfound freedom one night to begin pulling his intestines out of his anus until he was discovered and restrained.[38] Charles Bailiff, an epileptic patient who in 1880 suffered a series of fits which left him both energetic and violent, was removed to seclusion in a single room. The door of this room he promptly broke down, and he was placed in another, this time with his hands restrained by muffs. Sometime after 10pm that evening the night attendant made the decision to release him, as he was then quiet, and he promptly escaped through the window of his room. Bailiff got all the way to his own home, which he reached by travelling all night and arriving at 6.30 the next morning. He was wearing only his shirt and he 'willingly retuned' to Callan Park the next day.[39]

Not all the tasks allocated to the attendants were difficult or draining however: attendants regularly participated in amusements, escorting patients on picnics, trips to the circus or to see musical performances, and many played in the hospital's cricket team. Some limited travel was also available to staff: when patients were transferred between hospitals, senior attendants accompanied the men and women.

Most days were uneventful, with patients going about their jobs and amusements with no trouble and generally respecting the men who cared for them. Between 4.30 and 5pm each day the staff would dress for tea and dinner would be served either in the Dining Hall for calm patients or in the ward for those of a more energetic or violent disposition. Again, the cutlery would be counted back into the storerooms and patients would then retire for the night. In the summer patients went to bed at 7pm and in the winter 6pm. 'Privileged' or convalescent patients in the summer were sometimes allowed to stay up until 8pm.[40] Attendants would sleep in accommodation attached to the wards, and the night attendants would begin their vigils.

Like any private or public institution, Callan Park was subject to the usual laws in connection with deaths, practice and dismissal – all areas heavily involving attendants. Additional transparency of the workings of the state's insane hospitals had been brought in by Manning, and these were the

Official Visitors of New South Wales' asylums. Callan Park's first visitors were Sir Alfred Roberts, Dr J. C. Cox, and Mr Nugent Robertson – two 'medical men' and a 'barrister at law'.[41] In return for a small remuneration, their duties consisted of visiting Callan Park and inquiring into the care of the patients and the facilities. It was their role to advocate on behalf of the patients.[42]

Deaths of patients were passed to the Coroner.[43] In 1890 when Daniel Leary, a patient with symptoms of the 'general paralysis of the insane', drowned, there was an inquest. The Coroner found that even though Leary had not before shown suicidal tendencies at Callan Park, the attendants in charge of the working party he was a part of were not to blame as they had checked regularly on all patients under their care, and the place where Leary had entered the water had been partially obscured. A boy who was finishing off Leichardt Wharf witnessed the death, saying that he saw Leary jump into the water and wade about 30 yards from the shore and throw off his hat. Leary covered his own mouth with his hand, disappeared and reappeared several times, and then sank. The boy raised the alarm, and Leary's body was rescued and seen by one of the medical officers of the asylum who found he was dead.

The suicide of Dan Lynch, also in 1890, also attracted a coronial inquest. Again part of a working party, Lynch obtained permission from attendant Rennie to rest in the cricket shed. At the inquest Rennie maintained that Lynch had remained, as requested, in sight until twenty minutes past midday when Rennie found he could no longer see his charge. Lynch was discovered suspended from the rafters and Rennie was absolved from blame. The Coroner seemed to have been reluctant to find any attendant wanting in attention or action: after all, these attendants *were* looking after madmen – men who sometimes pursued death with a rigour elsewhere absent in their lives. It was impossible to watch *every* patient *all* of the time. But even in 1888 when James Ramsay killed fellow patient Frederick Heron by bashing him to death before breakfast in the airing court of their ward while in the presence of twenty other patients, and merely around the corner from both Skerritt and Mathison, neither attendant was found to blame.

Occasionally, complaints and accusations of cruelty were levelled at staff. Blaxland was not immune from this and in 1898 an article appeared in the *Cumberland Argus and Fruitgrowers Advocate* claiming an ex-patient of Callan Park had taken out a summons against Blaxland and a Dr Paton for 'alleged ill-treatment'.[44] Most complaints, however, concerned the attendants. Patients were a primary voice in making accusations. These were generally taken up and investigated by Blaxland and sometimes in combination with Manning. Mostly these claims were found to be false or exaggerated or the product of delusions. When confronted in 1884 with a complaint from William Crook (alias Williams) that attendant Latham had ill-treated him, it was with great exasperation that Blaxland recorded that 'Inquiry proved the matter to be a delusion, the patient stating that the injury took place four years ago in the Albury lockup'.[45] In 1882 William Dwyer, a serial escapee and a rather institutionalised young man, 'made some wholesale charges of cruelty against nearly all the Attendants of No 3 Ward'[46] to other patients while dressing one morning in April. Dwyer's main issue was the use of force used by several attendants in restraining a patient named Jowett who had been attempting to escape, an event Dwyer claimed he had witnessed. Dwyer said that attendant Skerritt had kicked Jowett with his knee, and that others, including attendant Sherack, had assisted in throwing Jowett to the ground. As part of the investigation, Jowett was questioned as to the truth of the story, and confirmed Dwyer's hyperbole. Dwyer's tales also showed concern for the 'lad named McKay' who he claimed had been manhandled into a chair after being 'carried by the arm alone'. Blaxland countered this accusation:[47]

> *The facts are that McKay is always very troublesome to dress, he kicks, bites, strikes and resists as much as he can, he is also possessed of ... chronic movements and on this morning he was dressed and carried by the two attendants who took him to a chair and just as they were putting him into it he jerked out of their hands into the seat, throwing out an arm and by spasmodically. The chair was a canvas easy one and McKay usually sits in it coiled up in a heap and kicks out or strikes when any one comes near him.*

Dwyer was not the only one: in the same year James Sewell decided to accuse attendant Barry of kicking,

> *... his skins, and showed where a small pieces of the cuticle had been knocked off, as a proof. He* [Sewell] *frequently makes unfounded charges against attendants and fellow patients and often gets into trouble with the latter on account of his aggressive and abusive nature. An investigation into the above complaint shows it to be utterly unfounded and apparently made maliciously with the view of getting Barry into trouble because Barry had to remove Sewell from the dormitory in the morning which he did by catching him by the shoulders and gently pushing him forwards.*[48]

Three months later, Blaxland had Sewell transferred to Gladesville.

Even the family of patients felt inclined to make complaints against the treatment of their loved ones, and mostly these were found after investigation to be either fantasy or exaggerations. The wife of John Burton Cox, a seriously violent patient in the final stages of the 'general paralysis of the insane' (or syphilis) and who spent his time at Callan Park destroying clothes, windows and furniture, and fighting with patients, complained that her husband was receiving rough treatment from the staff. She cited a bruise on her husband's arm to which Blaxland responded bluntly: 'On investigation I found evident exaggeration to say nothing of the gross mendacity of the complaint. There was no bruising or evidence of it, the swelling was a small abscess of the lymphatic gland which ... evidently resulted from a small abrasion'.[49]

But not every occasion involving his staff found Blaxland's support, and sometimes gross negligence or brutality was uncovered as existing in the wards of the hospital. Neither Blaxland nor Manning ever betrayed their own moral standing by whitewashing the conduct of their staff. Their investigations into issues were always swift and their decisions appear impartial. In fact, frequently Blaxland was obliged to reprimand his staff in order to maintain a high level of professionalism and care at Callan Park.[50] Warnings were Blaxland's first resort. In 1883 attendant Barry was severely reprimanded for 'extremely injudicious' treatment of Paul Guchery who sustained a cut eyelid and black eye after a confrontation with the attendant. Barry was described by Blaxland as having 'struggled' with Guchery after asking him to stop 'wrangling' with another patient, Scully. At this, Guchery removed his coat so as to continue the fight, and when Barry followed him 'to calm him' the two engaged in a struggle where they both fell to the ground. They had to be 'rescued' by a group of concerned *patients*. Blaxland warned Barry that 'any further trouble of the same sort would lead to his discharge'. Henry Webb's sprained ankle in 1886 ended in the reprimand of attendant Rex. Webb complained of rough treatment by two of his minders, Rex and Leddy. Leddy, having asked Webb to move from the mess room to the ward and been met with a refusal, called Rex for support. Webb struck Rex in the face and then the ribs, and Rex 'had to close with him and attempted to lay him down gently by tripping up his legs' but instead fell with him. Blaxland considered this a poor way of managing the situation and told Rex off. In 1887 attendant Blackburn was similarly reprimanded for the mishandling of Alexander Little and in the same year Carter, not noticing the gain of a black eye to one of his charges, and therefore failing to report it, was given an official warning.

Attendants were sometimes fined for their mismanagement.[51] Often the fine was used to pay to transport an escapee back to the hospital. In 1885 Nixon escaped by scaling a wall under the watch of attendant Welsh. Welsh, clearly at the end of his tether, preferred to resign than accept a reprimand and a fee. The year after when William Jones escaped after being left unattended at night in an unlocked ward, his attendant, Hughes, was fined by Blaxland for his carelessness. Later that year Hughes was fired for hitting a patient.

Blaxland regularly dismissed attendants who had either been careless or violent towards the patients of Callan Park. When attendant Dawes fell asleep on duty in 1892 he was sacked for leaving the patients unattended. In the parliamentary debate which discussed his removal from the asylum, other 'serious irregularities' with his conduct were also cited by Manning.[52] In October 1886 Amos Pearse made an unfounded complaint against attendant Keogh; a month later Keogh was summarily dismissed on the spot by Blaxland for drinking on duty. Blaxland recorded the event thus:

> *Attendant Keogh was reported last night by the attendant in charge of Ward ii (Rex) with being under the influence of liquor while on duty and with having ill-used a patient named Talbot. An investigation was made by me in conjunction with the Assistant Medical Officer (Dr Miles). An abrasion was found of the front of one of Talbot's wrists, who said it had been caused by Keogh and Rex's evidence borne out by several patients proved that Keogh had thrown the patient off a bed on which he was sitting. Attendants Rex, Towns and McIntosh all agreed that Keogh was under the influence of liquor. It appeared also that Rex remonstrated with Keogh about his treatment of Talbot when Keogh became abusive and passed his hand down Rex's face when the latter struck him in the face and a fight was only prevented by the intervention of the other attendants. When informed that his services were no longer required, Keogh became very abusive and threatening and in my opinion was under the influence of drink. This was about 2.30pm.*

Four days previously George Henry had also been instantly removed for kicking a patient. In 1887, George Miles, as acting medical superintendent of Callan Park while Blaxland took on Manning's role of Inspector General for some months, dismissed Rex after a scuffle with a patient named Patrick Clarke. Both Blaxland and Miles investigated the matter using the testimony of 'two rational patients' Williamson and Ferguson, who said that Rex had tried to remove some rubbish from the possession of Clarke and that when the latter had resisted, Rex had thrown him to the ground. Miles concluded that, 'Rex having been reprimanded twice before under somewhat similar circumstances he was today summarily dismissed'. Callan Park was not perfect – but even events which ended in dismissal had not gotten out of hand. Blaxland was easily provoked into action when he saw his staff behaving badly, which meant that staff not suited to their role were quickly weeded out and not allowed to fester and corrupt others. Any mistreatment of patients paled in comparison to the classic ideas of Victorian mental health care thriving in the public imagination. This was nothing compared to Reade's

Hard Cash hero, starved of sunlight and food, or Perceval's unhygienic and brutal treatment, chained to a wall.

But in 1900 Callan Park and its entire staff became the focus of a Public Service Board inquiry into the mistreatment of – interestingly – both patients *and* staff. Asylums had a reputation for being hotbeds of abuse, and suddenly Callan Park was in the spotlight, like Kew and Yarra Bend had been in Victoria some years ago. Blaxland had been medical superintendent at Balmain since 1881 and he faced his first wave of public and parliamentary scrutiny into the practice of his hospital.

The inquiry focused on the head matron, Miss Fairbairn, and her negligence in reporting the malpractice of one of the nurses, Bessie Smith. Smith was accused of administrating 'noxious ingredients' (a mixture of pepper, salt and water) to a patient and striking another with a mug in the face. Fairbairn was accused of failing to report these events to Blaxland, and of stealing fuel and wood from Callan Park for her own personal use. When nurse Annie Quilkey, abhorred with both Smith's cruelty and Fairbairn's lackadaisical approach to maintaining her staff, alerted Blaxland to these facts, Fairbairn was accused of dismissing Quilkey for her audacity. Blaxland was painted as a man no longer in command of his institution; even Whitling, the assistant superintendent, was under suspicion. His accountancy was reported as 'extravagant' and implied 'culpable negligence'.[53] Blaxland was later accused of bullying the nurses who had given evidence at the enquiry. The parliament was asked, 'Is the Prime Minister aware that a number of the nurses at the Callan Park Asylum who gave evidence at the recent inquiry by the Public Service Board ... are now being victimised by being removed for no stated reason, for their position at Callan Park to other asylums[?]'.[54] Another went on: 'the only reason for their removal is that they given umbridge to Dr Sinclair [Manning's successor as Inspector General] and Dr Blaxland'.[55]

The inquiry recommended Fairbairn be allowed to resign from her position as matron and cited her excellent nursing ability as contrasting to her woeful inability to head her nursing staff. It further advised the removal of Smith, and the investigation of Whitling's accounts by the chief inspector of public accounts. It went on to suggest that Quilkey be reinstated at another of the state's asylums, with compensation. Two female official visitors were also added, as per recommendation, to those visiting Callan Park – and Miss Parkes (the daughter of Henry Parkes) and Mrs Fitzsimmons (daughter of the late Dr Bedford) were rostered in.[56] Finally, and as the Colonial Secretary concurred with the Board's findings:[57] the largest change was made – Blaxland was removed from Callan Park and shunted sideways to Gladesville as the new medical superintendent there.[58] He joined his brother in law there, E. M. Betts, who was the assistant superintendent (that is, a clerk) there.[59] Parliament was instantly in uproar – was it not to Gladesville that the bullied nurses had been removed? Dr Sinclair said no.[60]

The medical superintendents of the state now began a game of musical chairs to accommodate the disgraced Blaxland's removal from Callan Park. Dr Williamson vacated Gladesville for Parramatta; Dr Godson left Parramatta and moved to the Kenmore Estate; Dr Ross left Kenmore and found Callan Park his new home. Mr Hepplewhite, formerly the clerk and foreman at Newington Asylum for infirm and destitute women – coincidently a house originally owned by Dr Blaxland's father – became the new Whitling, who retired.[61]

Dr Chisholm Ross, the new head of Callan Park, was a giant in the Lunacy Department at the time and regarded as a safe pair of hands. Originally from Inverell and one of ten children, like Blaxland he was educated after the Armidale School at King's. He received his medical degree from Edinburgh after leaving Australia in 1879.[62] Upon his return to the colony, he began his career in New South Wales asylums at Newcastle where he eventually became the medical superintendent there. He was Kenmore's first medical superintendent where, as described in his obituary, 'he planned the area and supervised the planting of trees. In doing that, he built for himself a monument that grows in beauty and power every year'.[63] Like Manning he was connected with the University of Sydney where he lectured and carried out some clinical work. After his time at Callan Park he became the government medical officer and then went into private practice in Macquarie Street. He was also a visiting medical officer at Reception House.[64] Ross died in 1934 after falling and injuring his shoulder while alighting from a tram. A month later and still in pain, he was discovered quite ill by his wife and passed away soon after. When he resigned from the New South Wales Lunacy Department in 1903 he was provided with a set of consulting room instruments, an album of images of Callan Park, a gold ring and an 'illuminated address signed by 174 members of the staff of the different hospitals for insane in the state'.[65]

Blaxland worked at Gladesville until he passed away in 1904. His demise was sudden. He died on a Sunday, after attending the hospital's church services and having done his usual rounds of the wards. At midday he was taken ill and died a little before midnight.[66] Blaxland was only fifty-two. He had reigned over Callan Park for a large portion of his life and spent much of his time away from his family, caring instead for the hundreds of patients in his asylums. When his corpse was removed from Gladesville and taken to the church for his funeral, his coffin would have passed by Manning's grave, only a few metres back from Victoria Road. Blaxland was not buried nearby his mentor, preferring to finally escape the asylum in death, and found rest in the Field of Mars Cemetery in Ryde. At his funeral nurses and attendants of Gladesville sang in the choir and his coffin was carried by further of his staff.[67] Two *In Memoriam* notices were placed in the *Sydney Morning Herald* after his death. The first was from the nursing staff of Gladesville. The second, and the more significant of the two, ran,

> *In fond and loving remembrance of Dr. Herbert Blaxland, late Medical Superintendent of Gladesville and Callan Park Hospitals, and Deputy Inspector-General of the Insane, who died at his residence at Gladesville, April 19, 1904. Inserted by united patients and ex-patients of Gladesville and Callan Park in respectful and grateful memory of his skill and kindness while under his care and trust.*[68]

5

THE ADMISSION PROCESS

There were three ways to gain access to New South Wales' still feared asylums in the late Victorian era.

The first and most common method was via arrest. Often those who exhibited signs of insanity did so publicly due to a lack of family support or even a house to call home. Many lunatics were homeless and friendless and were arrested after their symptoms indicated them to be a dangerous individual. Any sign of violence, directed personally or to others, was grounds for arrest. Sometimes, as the last resort of concerned family members, lunatics were directly deposited by family or friends with the police and simply abandoned at the police station. In either case – the arrest of a lunatic or the arrival of one at a police station – the police had several options to choose from as to what to do with the man or woman who was exhibiting symptoms of 'unsound mind'. Sometimes, of course, insanity was only discovered after arrest and while the inmate was installed in a cell.

In rural areas the options were more limited than in Sydney. Men and women arrested for lunacy and those discovered to be so while incarcerated were treated in a similar manner. Mainly, this consisted of managing the patient until transfer could be made to Sydney where the majority of asylums were. Often rural gaols had no facilities for caring for such people and often extreme violence was the result, with little done to reduce it. It is interesting to note, however, the care which was taken with these men and women. Even the most violent do not appear in the various *Punishment Books* attached to such gaols. An understanding seems to have existed that these were not normally-functioning human beings and therefore not deserving of punishment for their misbehaviour. When transport could be arranged, however, they were escorted to Sydney and either to the Reception House at Darlinghurst where they awaited processing and another transfer to the most appropriate asylum or, as more often occurred, were sent directly to an asylum. Either way, this usually would be one of the three main receiving hospitals for acute patients – Callan Park, Gladesville and Parramatta.

In Sydney there were more options for the police. In the case of those who had committed some crime in addition to obvious mental issues, they were placed in the Observation Ward at Darlinghurst Gaol for medical assessment. Many of these would then be transferred, along with their rural counterparts, to Reception House.

Arrest was not the only way however. Concerned loved ones could also apply for a Lunacy Petition or Lunacy Warrant and officially apply to have someone admitted to Reception House under a diagnosis of lunacy. The signatures of two doctors were required to officially certify one as insane, with the exception of those living in rural areas equipped with only one medical official. These patients with only a single signature on their blue lunacy petition could be admitted to Reception House, but until a second doctor signed they could not be admitted to one of the state's asylums proper.[1] These two doctors could not be related or in practice together or any relation to the medical superintendent of any New South Wales asylum. This method of committal was expensive however: the total cost of such a certificate amounted to a total cost of 10 guineas, a price the majority of people seeking state assistance to deal with their insane relative could not afford.

There was no law requiring the mentally unwell to be committed to the state's lunacy hospitals. If a family was in a position to support their loved one via private practice and this did not create any danger for either the patient or others, then there was no need to even register the patient with any governing body. As a result, Manning's yearly statistics as to the number of insane in the colony were based on those who were connected with the state hospitals and private madhouse at Cook's River, and not the wider – and usually richer – population. Committal to the state's asylums was generally for those of limited means in terms of support and/or money.

If families could not afford a warrant and the cost of the medical consultations needed for a doctor to sign the certificate, and did not wish to involve the police, there was a third option: simply arriving at one of the state's asylums, including Reception House, with the patient. This was called a 'Request'. In 1887 there was a distinct spike in the number of Requests observed by Blaxland at Callan Park. He wrote that 'Of the 193 admissions and readmissions [this year], no less than 103 were admitted under clause 8 of the Lunacy Act, by which both patients and their friends are saved the distress of appearing at the Police Court'.[2] These patients also avoided Reception House.

Reception House at Darlinghurst was Manning's invention, as a way to both classify and hold lunatics. It was opened in 1868. Importantly, it allowed insane inmates to be removed from gaols, which were poorly equipped to deal with them, while arrangements were made to place them in a hospital. The staff at Darlinghurst had several roles. Firstly, to care for the lunatic. This might include some limited treatment for mental disturbances as often men and women were brought in due to violence to themselves – sometimes an attempted suicide, for instance – and also physical care. Cuts needed to be cleaned, broken bones attended to, patients needed food, particularly if they had recently been homeless. Observation of the patient was also carried out, with notes made as to temperament, the use of any mechanical restraint, diet and sleep. Patients could be kept at the Reception House on remand for up to fourteen days, but most did not stay for longer than a week. Some, due to the effects of 'temporary insanity' usually brought on by excessive alcohol intake, were released as 'cured'. Most were transported in small groups to Sydney's various asylums. Their Reception House records often merely recorded 'sent to asylum'.

The police were often involved in the cases of lunatics before they received any medical help. In 1869, the same year his brother James Anlaby died, Legard was arrested – like so many of his fellow lunatic patients. An article detailing the event gives a terrible insight into Legard's life at this point:

WATER POLICE COURT – TUESDAY

(Before the Water Police Magistrate, and Messrs. Vess and Levey.) Frederick Legard was charged with breaking the windows of the premises occupied of Frederick Grant, in Darlinghurst Road. Prosecutor stated that he had promised to assist accused to get his clothes out of pawn. Last night accused came to prosecutor's house and demanded the fulfilment of this promise, but, as he was drunk, he was told to some again the following morning. The Bench fined accused 30s., and further remanded him for medical treatment in gaol.[3]

Legard had been drinking – suffering under the same vice as his father had – and had lost touch with the behaviour which came naturally to him as the educated son of a gentleman. Like Sir Thomas, Legard seemed also to have lost the ability to monitor his own finances. He was destitute, and increasingly violent. Darlinghurst Gaol was an ominous and terrifying place. A journalist touring the site in 1874 described his entrance to the facility:

A clangour of locks, bolts, and bars is the opening ceremonial of a visit to Darlinghurst Gaol, and the moment a stranger enters its precincts, his mind is impressed with the evidences round about of that force and physical restraint which constitute the basis of prison discipline. On the outer door there is a huge iron knocker, one stroke of which would almost awaken the dead; and on an experiment of its use being made, half a-dozen bolts fly back as if by magic, the door opens, remains so for a moment, and then rushes back noisily, to be barred and bolted as before. All is activity and watchfulness within... The left wing of this ... watch-house is used as an armoury, and the weapons there are placed in readiness for instant use, in case they should be so required.[4]

The Darlinghurst Gaol *Description and Entrance Book*[5] added that Legard was sentenced to twenty-one days imprisonment and was 'disposed of' on 31 May after having been treated, presumably, for injuries associated with the breaking of glass, in the hospital building within the gaol.[6] There is no indication in the records from Darlinghurst that Legard was supposed to be mentally unfit for discharge. Under 'occupation' is an acknowledgment of his highest qualification, Master of Arts. He was recorded as a Protestant who could read and write. Someone of Legard's education and family made him an unusual attendee of gaol.

When Legard was released he was homeless, often sleeping rough in the Domain. He assisted for some time in 1870 at a chapel in Manly, but otherwise depended on the kindness of friends and strangers for food and shelter. In 1871 a note in the *Sydney Morning Herald* notified a Frederick Legard of a letter awaiting him, but who might have been writing to him will remain a mystery. It is possible it was a message from his spinster sister Mary Anne, born only a year before Legard and foremost in his thoughts upon his eventual committal, where he named her as his next of kin and contact. Mary Anne died, unbeknownst to Legard in 1872, the year before his arrival at Reception House. Isabel and Henrietta, those barriers to his annuity, desperately needed at this point, were still alive on the other side of the world.

Homelessness saw a return to mental illness for Legard, who had staved off his insanity for over twenty years. In the time leading up to his arrest by the Water Police and conveyance to Reception House in 1873 he suffered from delusions, obsessive tendencies and was well known to the officers who patrolled the Domain. But he was not the young, energetic man as he had been in Charterhouse's kill-or-be-killed environment. He was sixty-one and had not the ability to survive as he once had. He had no one to support him and was without employment – the typical patient under Manning's tenure of the state's hospitals for the insane.

When Legard was picked up by the police and delivered to Reception House he was initially recorded as 'Frederick Lingard', which perhaps was indicative of the confusion during his initial admittance. He was diagnosed as suffering from 'slow onset' mania and was recorded as 'inclined to injure self or others' but was not suffering any injuries at the time. There is an emphasis in his papers that violence was a particular characteristic of his mania, but it was noted – wrongly – that his insanity was 'casual' rather than constitutional or hereditary. Legard was described as behaving well and sleeping little, and responding well to the shelter and food which Reception House afforded him. His delusions centred around the notion that he had been recently off catching bushrangers, and he was quoted as saying that he had come out of another world. Nine days later, Legard was transferred to Gladesville, where he named his deceased sister Mary Anne as his point of contact with the outside world. Legard had been alone in Sydney for some time: now, he had lost all communication with his family.

The medical staff at Gladesville recorded Legard as a married clergyman who had been suffering from chronic mania for the duration of ten days. It is unclear whether Legard himself provided this information – which in terms of his marriage was untrue – or whether the Gladesville staff merely assumed, perhaps upon the basis of his being a man of God. It was not recorded what particular event ended in his being deposited by the police at Reception House, but clearly there had been some public outburst which had prompted the police into action. The description of his having been 'queer for years' demonstrates perhaps his position on the radar of the local police in Sydney for some time. It also hints at the similarities between himself and Sir Thomas, who existed for some years in the society before his removal to the York Retreat. Legard certainly made an impression on the hospital staff: usually caring for uneducated labourers, and often foreigners, Legard was an intelligent English gentleman who had been living in Australia for over twenty years. The first entries in his *Medical Case Book* pages denote their interest:

> *He is an elderly man with sharpish features, grey hair and beard, and the indescribable 'something' about him which denotes the gentleman. He is very restless, flighty and locaucious, is vastly happy and contented with himself, claims everyone about him as relatives, is the victim of all sorts of fleeting delusions, and talks in the most random and nonsensical manner. He is at times* [illegible] *and mischievous but not violent and seems quite unable to appreciate his position. He takes food well.*

After the initial disturbance which landed him at Reception House, Legard calmed and began to act like the gentleman he said he was. The staff were quickly informed of his family: 'It appears that he belongs to the Yorkshire family of Legards, is a Clergyman of the Church of England and a Graduate of Cambridge; that it is several years since he officiated as a Clergyman'.

In the first few weeks of Legard's stay at Gladesville, where he was sent prior to Callan Park's opening, and during the time he was under close observation he was described as 'manageable' but 'interfering'. He was well-spoken and helpful, but compelled by strong fancies to put buttons in his ears, and was prone to boisterous and bossy behaviour, particularly when it came to his interactions with other patients. This is easy to understand: Legard was of a higher class than most of his fellow patients; he was educated and refined. For someone 'unable to appreciate his position' it would be natural for him to assume a position of higher status when dealing with his fellows. He did not always display this supremacy however: for such an Englishman, cricket was a favourite past time and he regularly participated in games with other patients. Legard was described in his file as 'a favourite with all the children in the district and is always surrounded with them whenever he goes to the cricket paddock' – an activity which he continued to pursue at Callan Park under Blaxland.

A year later, in August 1874, he was described as in excellent health and having had no 'attacks' of noise or excitement as previously characterised him. His contact with children and lack of violence generally, along with his willingness to assist in the wards and the office, was evidence of his better mental health. But Legard's illness made him inconsistent in this regard: by November of the same year he was a recluse in the hospital, spending 'his whole time at arithmetic'. The following March he was happy to work, but again by May, he refused to assist and went obsessively back to his books. For the staff at Gladesville this obsessive behaviour would have been a clear indication of Legard's tenuous grip on mental stability and systematic of his unwillingness or lack of ability to care for himself if discharged. Viewed as most probably a chronic patient unlikely to ever be removed from care, in

May 1876 Legard was transferred as one of the first forty-four to Garryowen House at Callan Park.

Once a patient arrived at his asylum he would be admitted to the Admissions Ward (Ward Four – or Ward Seven for women) and would undergo further observation. He would be accompanied by a large sheet of paper with notes as to his past history if any was known, along with details of his treatment at Reception House. Any property he had had on him at the time of his admission to Reception House would be noted on his form. This usually consisted of small amounts of money, matches, knives. This information would be copied into his file and after a few weeks he would be transferred to the most appropriate ward in the hospital. The master-in-lunacy, Arthur T. Holroyd, would then investigate the patient's financial situation and look into any property he might own and, in the case of there being no relatives available to liaise with, he would begin his watch over the patient's finances. If the patient could contribute to his care, then funds were withdrawn at regular intervals from his accounts. If the patient held property, the master-in-lunacy controlled the leases. The master-in-lunacy's role was two-fold: to collect payments from patients but also to look after the patient's interests. Before the role was created in 1879, after the passing of the 1878 Lunacy Act,

> *... no one was in a position to deal with the estate of an insane patient except by going through the expensive form of taking out a writ* de lunático inquirendo, *and having a committee appointed. But now, under the 105th section of the present Act, it is enacted that the Master-in-Lunacy shall take care of, and collect and administer under its provisions, the property and estates of all insane patients.*[7]

Holroyd was rather mercenary in his collection of payments: they were always on time, and even when patients' families fell on hard times, he ensured some – even a small – payment was made. The moment Legard was able to contribute to his care, due to the deaths of his last sisters, Holroyd immediately began to charge him.

Importantly, no matter how a patient arrived at hospital, they were examined by at least two doctors on their journey there. Manning in the meantime would personally review the Lunacy Papers and, as previously discussed, would sometimes void certificates if they were problematic and liberate the sane person. Thus 'inconvenient' wives, husbands and other family members could not just be shut away in Manning's hospitals. If they were not mad, there was no place for them: no one at Callan Park profited by keeping a sane patient within the asylum.

There were only a limited number of mental conditions regarded as requiring committal in the 1800s. These could be sorted into three categories: mania, melancholia and dementia. Mania and melancholia retain the same broad definitions today, but dementia in the Victorian era had broader connotations including the dullness of wits, confusion, along with a lack of animation and reduced understanding. The three disorders were caused by a range of factors, namely: isolation (from home-country, and friends and family, and which was particularly prevalent in immigrants and those in rural areas), hereditary taint, congenital mischief, intemperance, sunstroke (a cause particular to Australia, and a new factor for the British-educated doctors to combat), injury to the head, epilepsy, fever, ill-health, destitution and old age.[8] Thus the wide range of mental disorders we recognise today were reduced to a choice of three: extreme and energetic high spirits, extreme depression, and non-understanding, and all thought to be caused by a range of both legitimate and strange factors.

Treatment for these diseases consisted primarily of the principles of Moral Therapy, but in the same way that some restraint was often used, so were some drugs. Investigation into the drugs prescribed by Callan Park's dispenser in the 1870s and 1880s has yielded some surprising results.[9] Other than sedation through injections of morphine and potassium bromide, patients did not receive any medical treatment for delusions or hallucinations. In extreme cases, patients were secluded in single rooms until fits passed. In the case of mania and melancholia the best that doctors could find was cannabis indicti and this offered only limited results. In the case of hypochondriacally-minded patients, sometimes placebos were provided. One patient in the 1880s was given a draught – a tonic taken in one swallow – of a very weak mixture of potassium bromide and water, to calm him.

The bulk of prescriptions made for patients were for much more banal complaints: sore throats and coughs, urinary tract infections, rheumatism and reduced appetite. Castor oil was regularly given to patients suffering from constipation, and sometimes in conjunction with opium for pain. Antimony tartrate was also a powerful emetic used. In the case of one patient who suffered from prolonged and severe epileptic fits, he was given an enema consisting of a mixture of castor oil, turpentine and water during a particularly long seizure of three hours duration. This use of 'heroic medicine' – the archaic belief which also encouraged the bleeding of patients as the way to health – is an interesting aberration from the otherwise fairly enlightened Callan Park. In this man's notes, it was written that after his bowels moved the treatment was successful in ending the fit.[10]

Magnesium sulphate (Epsom salts) were often prescribed for cramps and muscle soreness. For stomach aches belladonna was used, along with hot poultices and sodium bicarbonate. Dry mouth was combated with lemon juice. Quinine sulphate appears often as a reducer of fever and to still cramps. Anaemic patients were given ferric sulphate, and tonic of digitalis was provided as a heart stimulant. Some of the shorthand in the patients' files describes 'in-house' mixtures known only to the doctors at Callan Park in the 1880s. But even without these, the dispenser's notes in the files paint a rather helpless picture. Drugs which are easily supplied today to manage depression and mood swings did not exist. It is interesting to note, however, that without these medicines, which often limit the life of twenty-first century sufferers due to kidney or liver disease associated with the prescription, lunatics in this time tended to live extensively long lives. Cared for with shelter, cleanliness and regular food, many lived into their seventies and eighties.

In 1894 a letter arrived at Callan Park for Blaxland from a James Digby Legard RN, who was Frederick Legard's nephew and the son of his brother James Anlaby. A few months previously Frederick had taken the time to write to his brother James Anlaby. The letter had been passed to James' son – James

Digby – due to his decease some decades previous.

The tone of the return letter from James Digby Legard, whose image even today hangs in the National Portrait Gallery in London, is saddening. It is interrogative and clearly conveys his complete lack of interest in the Callan Park patient, who does not seem to have had a single visitor in the three decades he lived at the Balmain hospital before his death. Coming quickly to the point, James described Frederick's letter as 'so incoherent it was impossible to form any opinion as to the identity of the writer', making no allowance for his uncle's state of mind or advanced age. There is something very mercenary in this letter too: James gives no hint at happiness in being thus contacted by his aged uncle, now in his eighties. In fact, the response appears entirely fiscally-motivated. At the end of the letter, James made his point. His reason for bothering to reply was simple: to ascertain 'the identity of the recipient of [the] annuity' then being paid to Frederick from James' own estate. James' doubts as to Frederick's identity were made cruelly clear, adding that 'all his [Frederick's] brothers and sisters have been dead some years and none of them lived to such an advanced age'.

Notes in the margins of a copy of James' letter, initialled by Blaxland and intended as a basis for Manning's reply to James Digby, indicate Frederick Legard's advanced age and increasing feebleness, and do not seem to doubt at all the identity of the old patient. One, entirely ignoring the possibility that the patient was not who he claimed to be, reads, 'He is very demented now and is extremely poor in physical health though still able to be up and about. He has had one or two [illegible] apoplectic seizures and will not in all probability survive the coming winter'.

But the patient called Frederick Legard *did* survive the winter, and he was most *certainly* who he said he was.

Legard was described in his file at this time as 'very delusional' but 'in fair health considering his age'. By 1896 he was confined to bed and being treated for an aortic murmur. Finally, on 24 June 1897 he died in his bed from 'senile decay'. In all his time at Callan Park and there is nothing to suggest his family ever made the slightest attempt to communicate with him. This last child of Cecilia and William Legard, loved best by his father and seemingly despised by his mother, continued to receive his annuity until his death, despite the efforts of James Digby. Like so many patients, Frederick died without leaving a will, and was buried in one of the far reaches of Rookwood Cemetery under the gum tress and amongst the very-Victorian ferns. There were likely no mourners at his funeral and his headstone has been wiped clean by time.

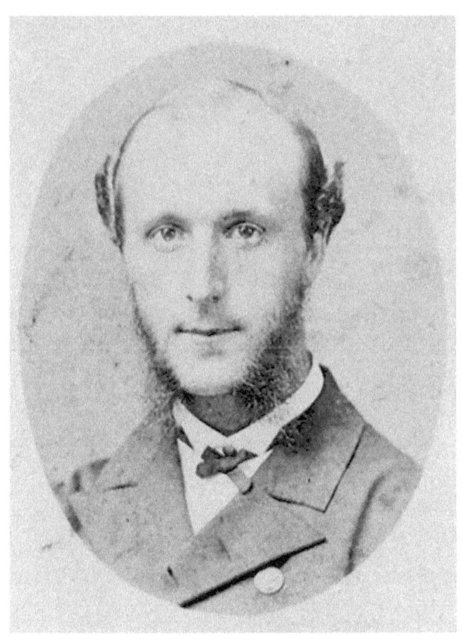

Left

1. Dr Frederic Norton Manning, the first Inspector General of the Insane in New South Wales, as a young man

Dr Norton Manning, c.1862–6, photographer Bradley & Allen. Call Number P1 / 1105, State Library New South Wales

Below

2. Dr Herbert Blaxland, medical superintendent of Callan Park Hospital for the Insane (1881–1900)

Faulkner John Blaxland photographs, drawings, print and realia relating to the Blaxland and Norton families, 1790–c.1970. Call Number PXE 1216 – Box 2, State Library New South Wales

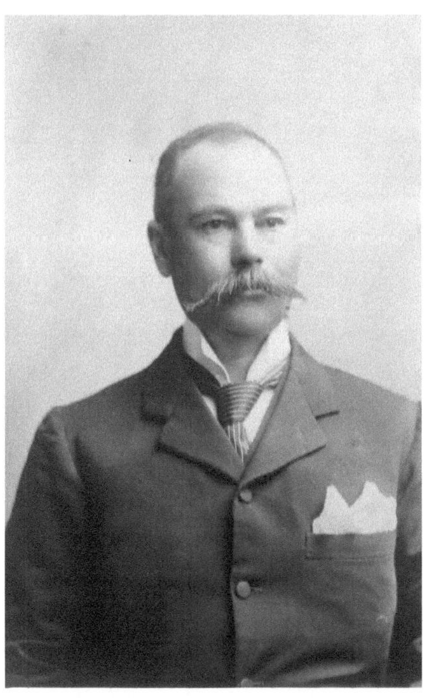

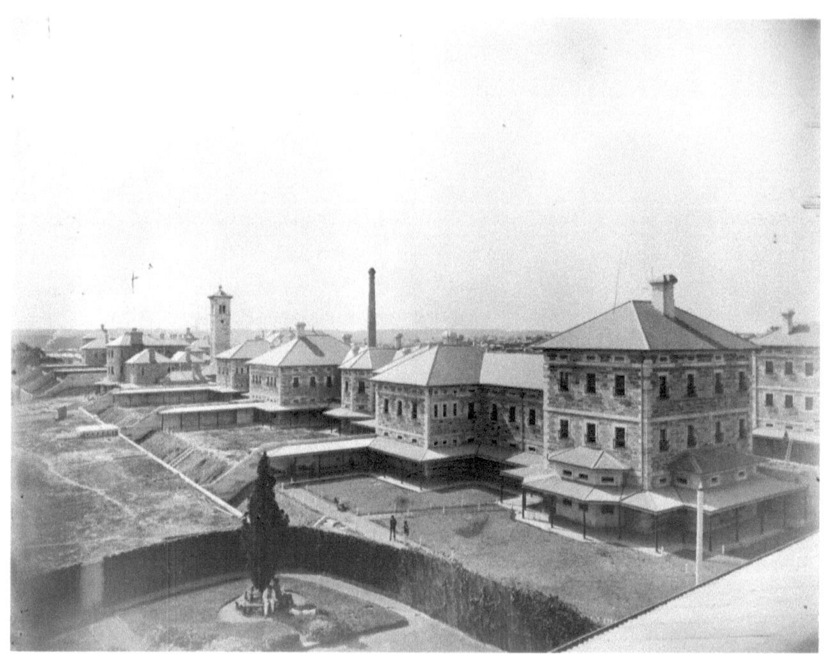

3. The private courtyard at Garryowen, with patients relaxing under the tree, overlooks the back of the Kirkbride Complex
SRANSW: 'View of Callan Park Hospital, Rozelle (NSW)' [4481_a026_000138]

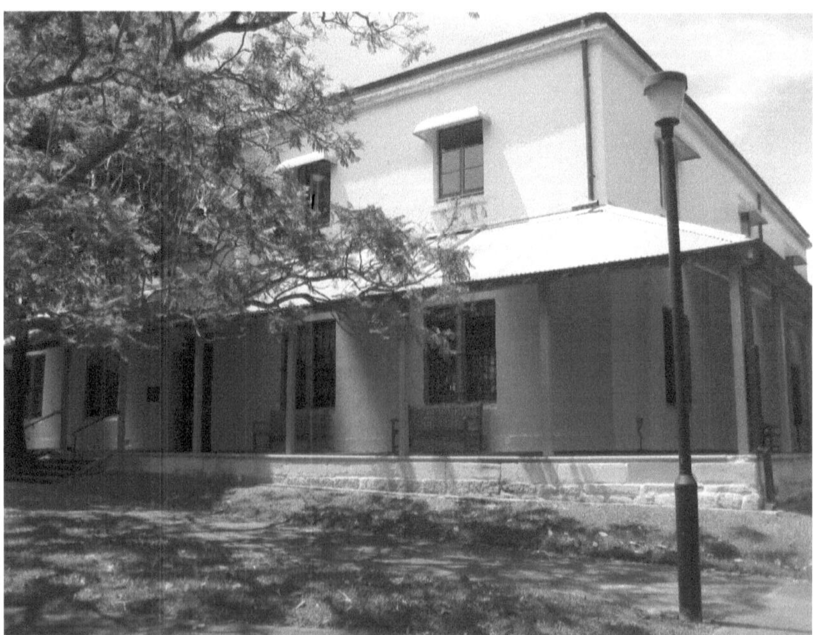

4. Garryowen House today, home to the New South Wales Writers' Centre
Photograph by S Luke (2017)

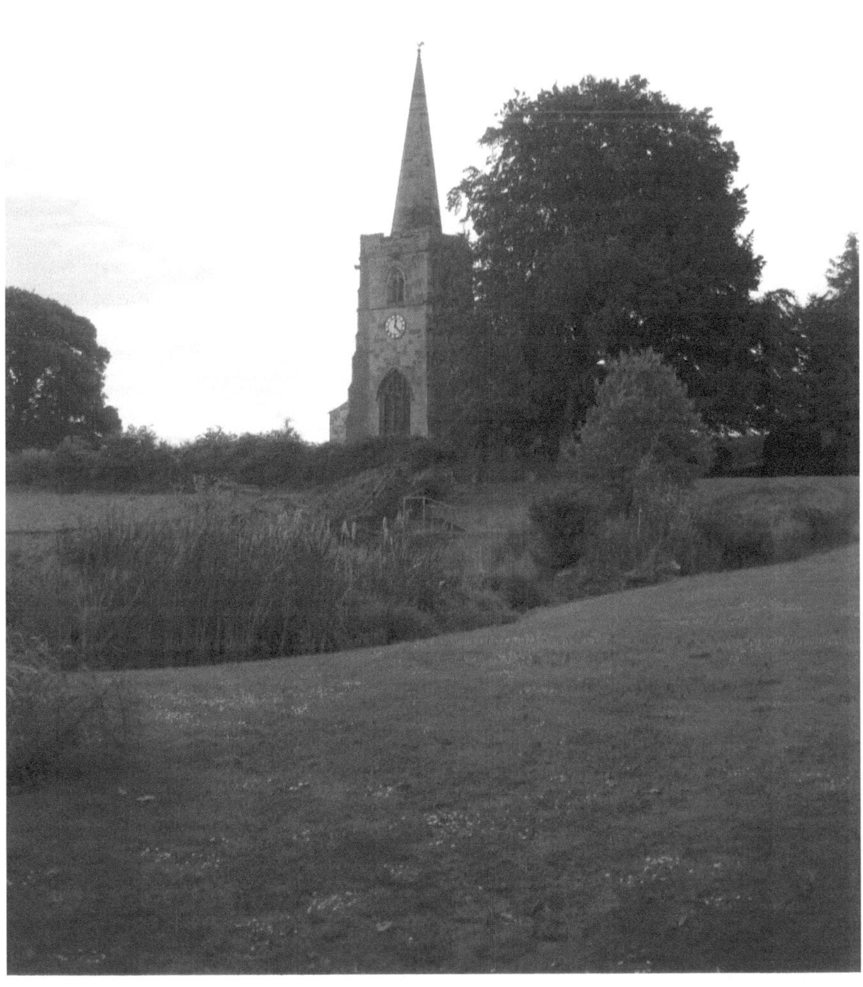

5. St Nicholas Church at Ganton, Yorkshire, where Frederick Legard was reverend before he moved to Australia
Photograph by S Luke (2016)

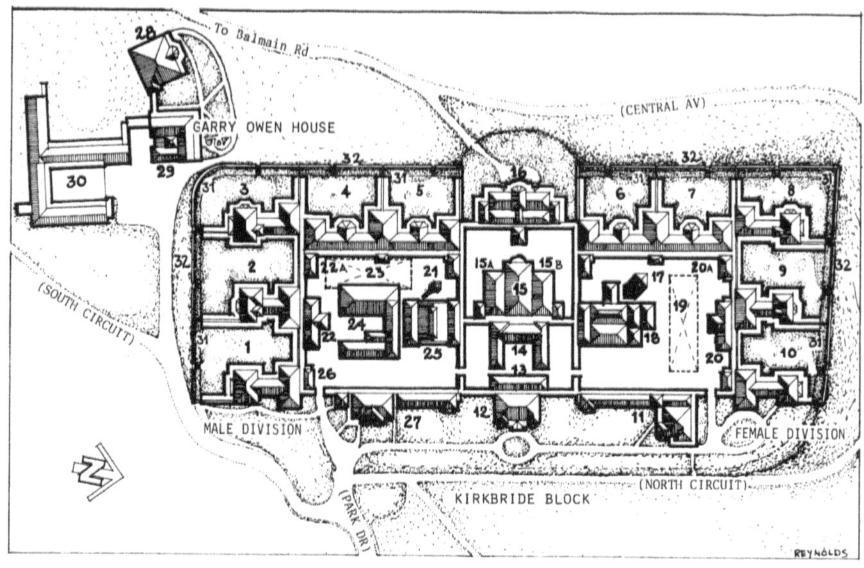

6. Map showing the layout of the wards at Callan Park, including the private ward for men at Garryowen House. The private female wards, which were located just off Central Avenue, are not shown on this map

Key:

1 Ward One (for convalescent men)
2 Ward Two (for violent and refractory men)
3 Ward Three (for intermediate men)
4 Ward Four (for admissions and acute men)
5 Ward Five (hospital ward for men)
6 Ward Six (hospital ward for women)
7 Ward Seven (for admissions and acute women)
8 Ward Eight (for intermediate women; contains a basement underneath the ward)
9 Ward Nine (for violent and refractory women)
10 Ward Ten (for convalescent women)
11 Medical superintendent's residence
12 Administration block
13 Store
14 Kitchen
15 Recreation hall / chapel
15a Male dining hall
15b Female dining hall
16 Medical Officers' Wing
17 Water tower
18 Laundry
19 Underground tank
20/20a Planned female bath house site / actual site
21 Boiler chimney stack
22/22a Planned male bath house site / actual site
23 Underground tank
24 Stables and workshops (now demolished)
25 Boiler house and engine room
26 Mortuary (demolished)
27 Dispenser's residence and chief attendant's residence
28 Extension to Garryowen House for private male patients
29 Garryowen House
30 Temporary weatherboard wards (demolished)
31 Boundary of airing courts, including ha-has
32 Perimeter wall

'Hospital for the Insane, Callan Park: 1880–1885' in P. Reynolds, 'Garry Owen and Callan Park, The story of Rozelle Hospital, Lilyfield: 1819–1984', *Leichhardt Historical Journal* No. 14 (1985), p. 62

Image courtesy of Inner West Council Library Services, Original Materials Collection, Inner West Council Community History and Heritage Collection

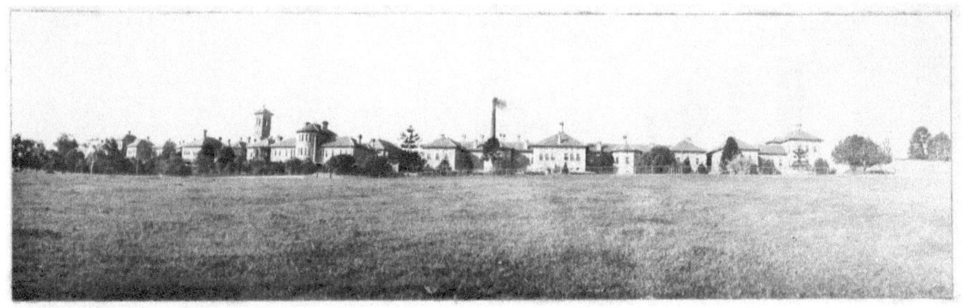

7. Callan Park's imposing skyline. Note the clock tower, which never received its clock faces

Above and figures 8–13:

'Callan Park, A Great State Institution', *Sydney Mail*, 12 August 1903, photographs by Alfred Small [Photographs of Callan Park Mental Hospital, 1903], Call Number PX*D 241, State Library New South Wales

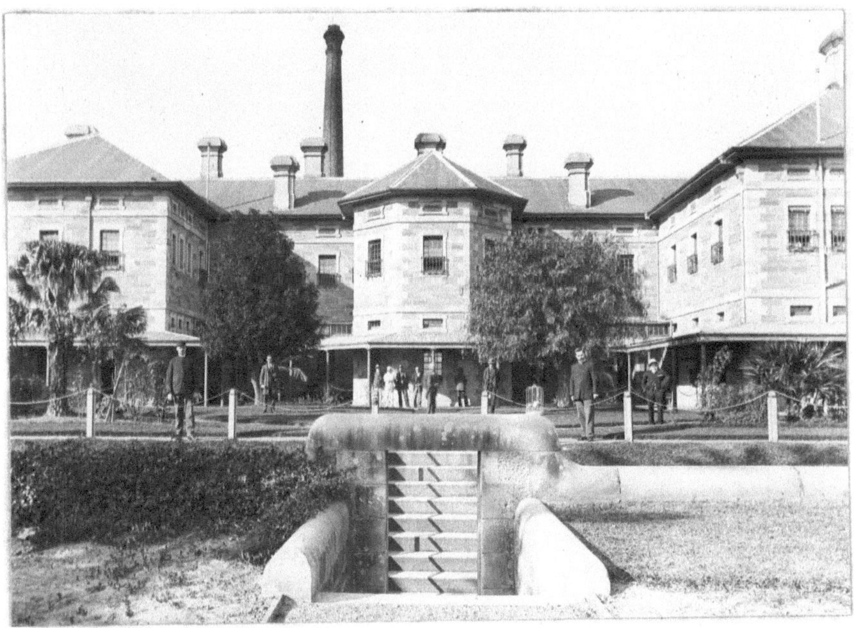

8. Attendants, nurses and patients outside one of the Kirkbride wards for men. Note the caged pet bird on the step – one of the many pets donated to the hospital

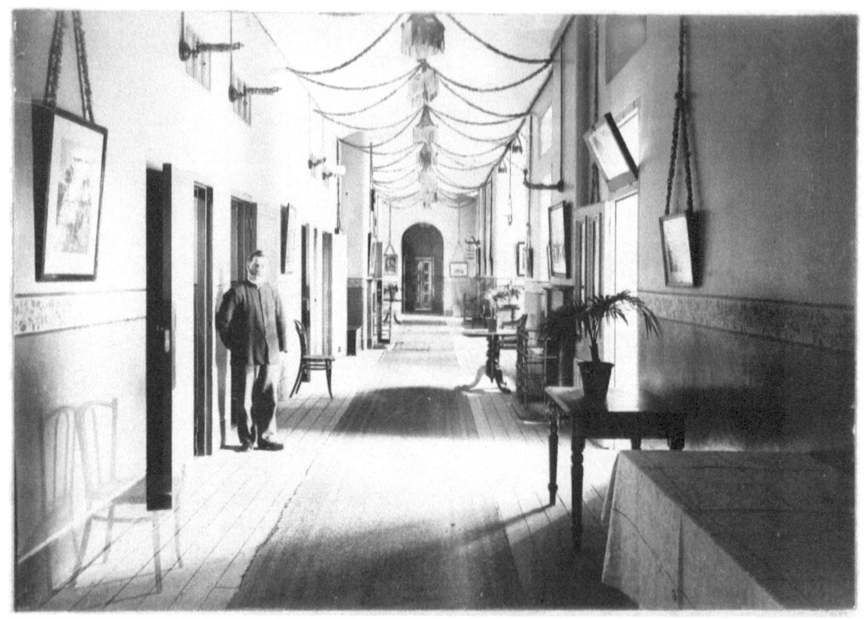

9. Single rooms and a homely day corridor in the Kirkbride Complex, with a male attendant on duty

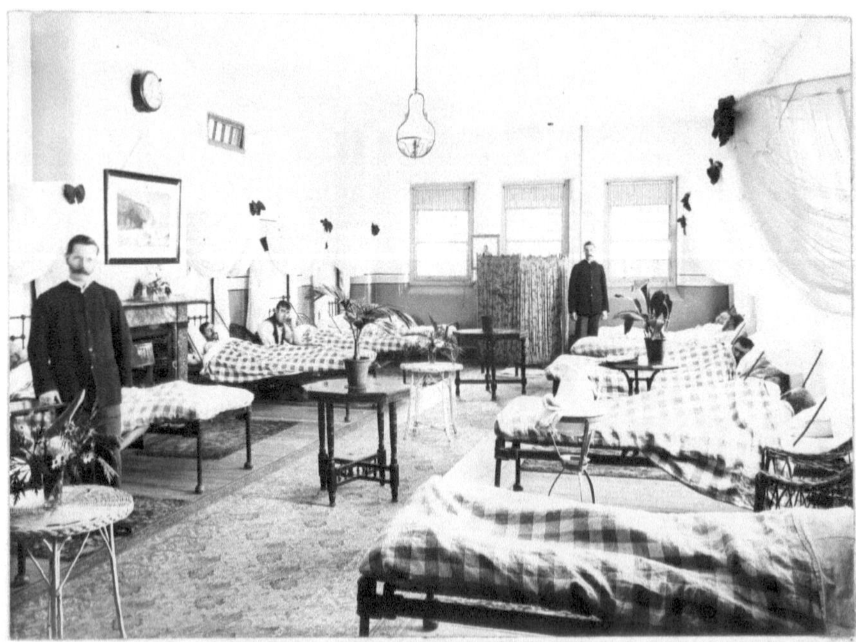

10. The interior of one of the male wards in the Kirkbride Complex, probably a dormitory in the Hospital Wing (Ward Five)

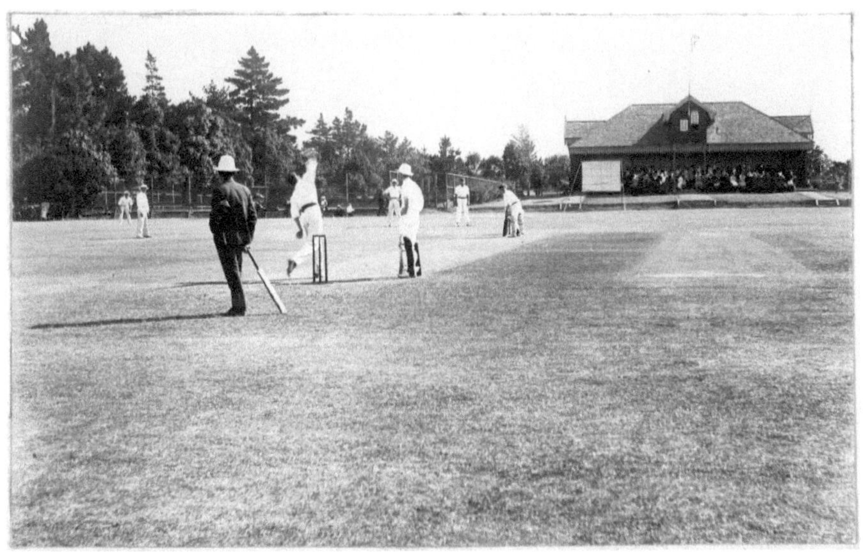

11. A game of cricket. The handsome pavilion was designed by an early patient, possibly John Cane. The tennis court is just visible on the left

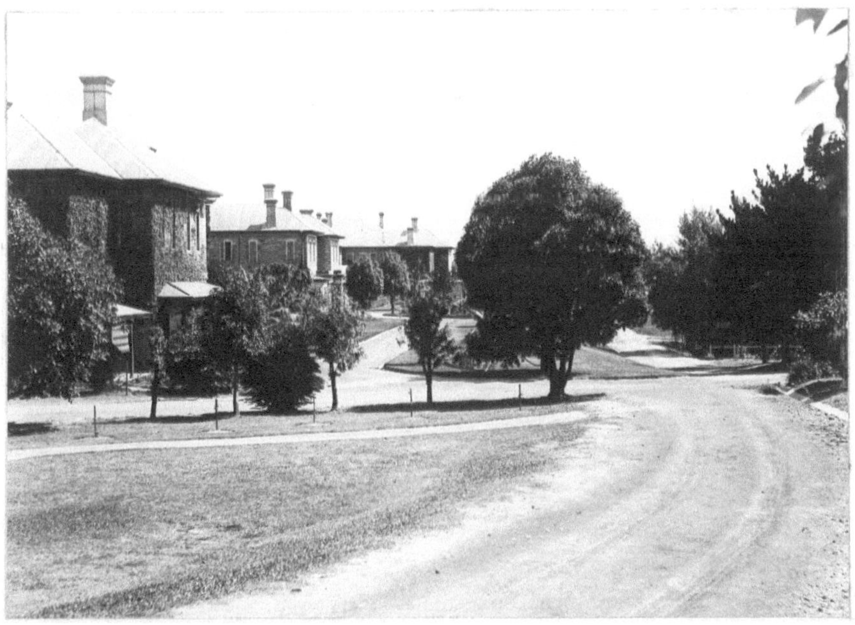

12. A view of the drive towards the Administration block in the Kirkbride Complex

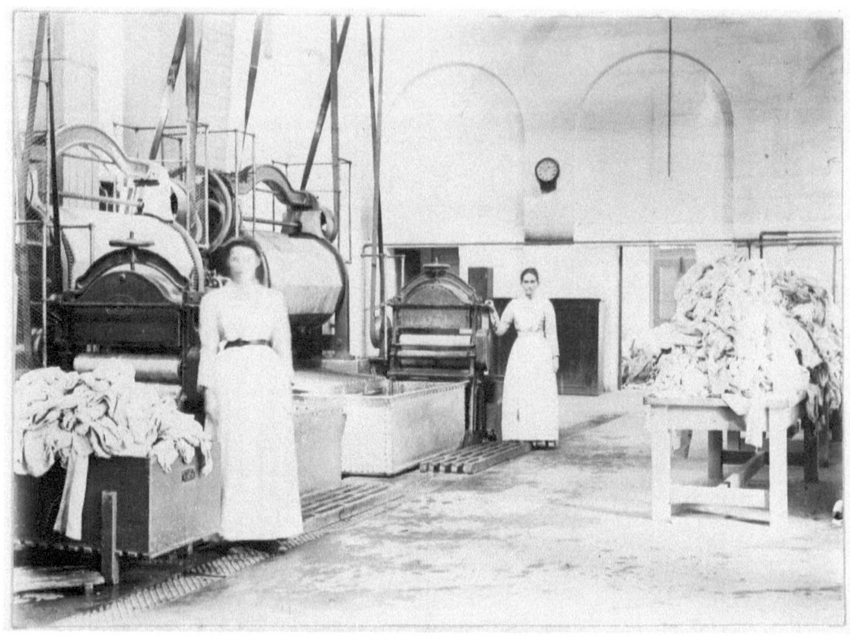

13. Laundresses in Kirkbride's laundry

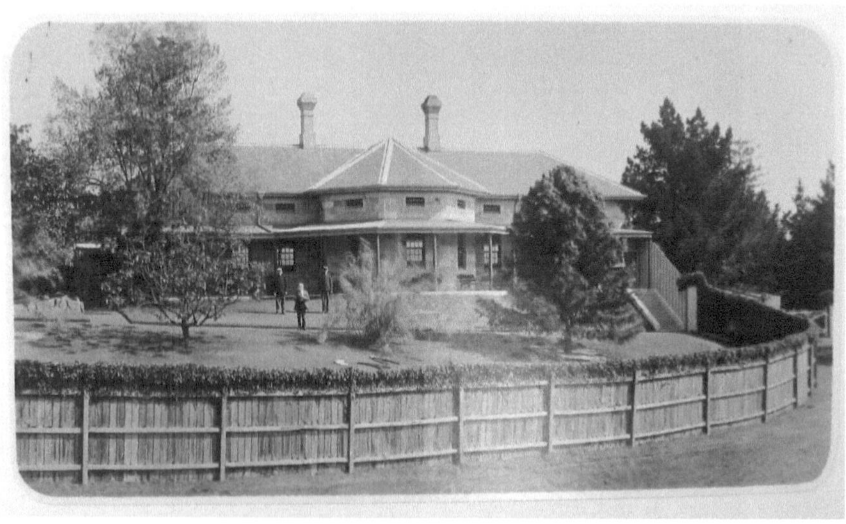

14. The private cottage for men, connected to Garryowen, opened in 1888

Family and holiday album, 1899–1908, photographed by Arthur D. Whitling. Call Number PXE 917, State Library New South Wales

PART TWO
THE PATIENTS

6

MEN VERY FAR FROM HOME

In November 1888 a disturbing notice appeared in the *Newcastle Morning Herald and Miner's Advocate*: 'An escaped lunatic from Gladesville, an Italian, was recaptured at Auburn. He stated he was an Italian prince.'[1] Nine years later this 'Italian Prince' was transferred to Kenmore as one of its first, and chronic, patients. He lived there until his death in 1940 at eighty-six years of age. First committed to Gladesville when he was only twenty-four, in 1878, and one of the four groups of twelve transferred in 1879 to the ranks of Garryowen, Italian Fillipo Parcelli spent almost his entire life in New South Wales' asylums.

A lifetime in one place might very well be a disturbing prospect to anyone – and even more so if one's home is full of terror and brutal treatment at the hands of inhumane 'carers'. Was Parcelli's 1888 escape a cry for help against humiliating, dehumanizing treatment or merely the confusion associated with one in the throes of a deep mania?

Fillipo Parcelli (known variously as Parcellie, Tomassini, and either Phillipo or Fillipo)[2] was born in 1854 in Italy and lived there, working as a clerk, until his early twenties. He was moderately-well educated, and like Legard could both read and write. He was five feet seven inches tall, a slight man with a dark complexion, and had black hair with hazel eyes and a scar on his forehead. Like so many other Europeans in the 1800s, Parcelli saw a journey to the new British colony of Australia as a new start and an adventure. As there is no evidence to suggest that Parcelli was of unsound mind either before departing Europe or that any symptoms became clear during the long ship journey, we must assume that his presence in Australia was not because his family wished to be rid of him. He arrived in the major Queensland port of Maryborough, a little north of Brisbane, in January 1877, after having departed Hamburg late in 1876.

In the proceeding eighteen months after his first moments in Queensland, Parcelli would marry, be thrown into gaol and be committed to Gladesville Hospital for the Insane.

Either unwilling or unable to find work in his preferred profession, Parcelli found employment as a labourer in Queensland before moving to New South Wales. It was possible that this work – both physically demanding and in a more rural setting than he was used to – contributed to his decline in mental health. Manning's ideas[3] on the power of isolation from family, friends, normal routine and one's home country, state clearly that culture shock could tip any rational being into insanity, particularly in the dry and unrelenting heat of Australia. Working as a common labourer was no doubt a slight drop in status for young Parcelli, and without the support of family, he may have encountered a deep homesickness. Additionally, a pre-existing condition could easily have been exacerbated by his new work and environment. Either way, Parcelli's first few months in Australia cannot have been easy.

But relief came and more than likely kept his symptoms at bay: before he moved to New South Wales Parcelli married Fernandine Louise Jesine Holbessen. Together they moved to Young in New South Wales, rich gold country and a town with fertile farming land. Parcelli supported himself and his new wife by continuing to labour in Young, and their life together was quiet until August 1878 when he was arrested for vagrancy. Possibly a sign of the breakdown of his marriage, Parcelli had taken it upon himself to write to each eligible lady in Young with an offer of matrimony. This was too much for the small community of Young to bear and Parcelli was arrested and incarcerated in Young Gaol for his misdemeanour. Upon his delivery to the gaol, it was noted that two fingers on Parcelli's right hand were broken, possibly an indication of his increasing violence. Parcelli was sentenced to three months hard labour.

It was not long before the warder at Young Gaol realised that Parcelli was not well. During his initial days in the gaol he assaulted his keeper, was suicidal and noisy – a characteristic which was to describe the decades of care ahead of him – and he was continually attempting escape, a clear indicator that he was not happy at his confinement. It was quickly obvious that this inmate was not of rational mind. The staff at the gaol were compassionate: despite this misbehaviour Parcelli was not 'punished'[4] for flouting the rules as any ordinary prisoner would have been. Parcelli was quickly transferred out of the gaol – serving less than a month of his sentence – and taken to Reception House in Darlinghurst, Sydney.

The journey from Young to Sydney was a long one and Parcelli not the most accommodating of patients. He was described as 'noisy and violent' and to ensure his own and others' safety, was transported in the end by the wearing of a camisole to restrain him. At this point it is unclear if his wife went with him to Sydney. Certainly, at Gladesville where he was admitted after a short stay at Reception House, his wife was not listed as his next of kin. Instead a Mr Fitzgerald, the consular agent for Italy, was listed as his contact. In the Gladesville *Medical Case Books* Parcelli was listed as single – but, again, whether this was the assumption made by an employee, or the information provided by a lunatic, there is no way of knowing. Further, there is no indication that his wife visited him at any of the hospitals where he was cared for in his life. There was, however, a child – Arthur W. Parcelli – born to a Fernanda and Phillipo Parcelli in Sydney in 1879 and this suggests that Fernandine did follow her husband to Sydney, though whether she stayed in contact with him is unclear from his medical files.

Gladesville classified Parcelli as suffering from mania, given his energy and violence. He was described as being afflicted by frequent outbursts of maniacal excitement during which he would 'demand his liberty'. In addition, he was continually noisy and very troublesome in his ward. There is no doubt that Parcelli was housed in Ward Two at Gladesville – which used the same numbering system as Callan Park: Ward Two was reserved for the most violent and aggressive 'refractory' patients, of which Parcelli was most certainly one. Upon admission, the doctors at Gladesville further noted his coated tongue, a slight conjunctive congestion and that he complained of a headache bad enough that if he had a razor on him he would happily cut his throat to escape the pressure on his skull. On examination 'during his quieter intervals' he was able to give 'a very connected account of his past history' which included, he said, the attempt by a stranger to poison his whiskey while in Young. Suspicions concerning poisoning were a common feature of the paranoia experienced by many patients in Australian hospitals. As a result of this fear, Parcelli was unwilling to take medicine prescribed him, scared of further poisoning attempts and as a result did 'not make any improvement' for some time. Frequent violent episodes also characterised his time at Gladesville: kicking doors down when in seclusion, tearing off his clothes and jumping around, screaming incoherently. In contrast, sometimes he was silent, sullen and solitary. To quote his Gladesville medical files, he appeared 'to be very insane'.

Today Parcelli might be diagnosed with something along the lines of bipolar disorder, but in the nineteenth century he was 'manic' and the staff paid to deal with him focused their efforts merely on containing him when violent. But Gladesville was overcrowded and Parcelli, often a handful to look after, was transferred to Callan Park in October 1879 with a number of equally maniacal men: Henry Jollis, a twenty-seven-year-old boot finisher; Amos Pearse, a fifty-seven-year-old tailor; William Andrews, a twenty-nine-year-old labourer; and Alexander Clubb, a twenty-nine-year-old plasterer. Mr Fitzgerald at the Italian consulate, and not Parcelli's wife, was notified of the change of location in Parcelli's treatment. In the grand tradition of the understating of patients' conditions which seemed to go on whenever inmates were transferred from Gladesville to Callan Park, Parcelli was described as 'not a troublesome patient' in the paperwork which accompanied him to Garryowen. The sheet added that 'his expression is somewhat wild, his temper variable, he is often angry at his detention' and finished with 'he has occasional attacks of noise and excitement'.

In December, when Callan Park held just under 100 patients, Parcelli was involved in two serious incidents. The first was when he struck one of the attendants of Ward Two, housed in the weatherboard extension beside

Garryowen. Attendant Skerritt's injuries must not have been severe, as they were not recorded, but Parcelli was secluded for an hour for his behaviour. Ten days later, Parcelli joined in a pre-meditated attack on Skerritt and other Ward Two attendants with three other patients, Samuel Payne, a paranoid and melancholic man, the aged Frederick Legard who was more eccentric than insane, and William Clancy.[5] Clancy was a thirty-six-year-old butcher suffering from dementia caused by intemperance. After having threatened violence to one of his five children he had been committed by his wife. During his stay at Callan Park he was diagnosed with *petit mal,* small epileptic fits. He was described as manageable but, like Parcelli, sometimes angry at his detention. In 1890 he was re-diagnosed with chronic mania and died suddenly six years later of a cerebral haemorrhage. This interesting group 'attacked' the attendants, wrote Dr Scholes, and were secluded for an extensive four and a half hours from 1.30pm to 6pm, an hour before bedtime.

There are two reasons why these men were secluded. Those of the sensationalist Victorian mindset would naturally assume that such a response spoke of rigid punishment and Scholes' wish to assert his authority through rough treatment and isolation. But what is far more likely is that these men posed a serious risk to not only the staff and other patients, but also themselves. Seclusion was not conducted in airless stone cells but light, airy rooms with a view outside – or, sometimes, in the patient's own single room if he had been allocated one. It is unclear whether these men were secluded in their own single rooms or in the padded rooms built to contain such an outburst. Parcelli was labelled 'very dirty' at times in his file which generally was the term used to describe a patient who was unable to control his own bodily functions. It is for this reason that it is highly likely that Parcelli slept – and was secluded – in one of the panelled rooms, which would have been easier to clean than one of the regular single rooms. But the question over the level – if any – of brutality used to subdue and then seclude these four men, is more difficult to answer. Did Skerritt twist an arm a little more heavily that day than he might normally have done? Did any of his fellow attendants throw any punches – even if it were in defence? Were any of the four thrown to the floor or treated in any way than men out of their minds ought to be?

Scholes, Blaxland, Ross – they never avoided vivid descriptions of fights and other incidents of violence. They did not discriminate between abuse wielded by staff or patients – all was recorded, good or bad, in the *Medical Journals*. From the report written up, Scholes implied that the violence was all from the patients, and staff moved only to calm, not to take revenge.

By March 1880 Parcelli was described as being 'rather quieter of late and better behaved': the excitement of the rapid influx of new patients into Garryowen had abated and life at Callan Park could proceed without novelty or disturbance. That Parcelli could read means that he might have made use of the library at Callan Park during his more placid intervals. His labouring skills may have allowed him enjoyment in working the gardens or caring for the pets. But Parcelli's state of mind was in constant change and in May, while in the airing court of Ward Two one day, he suddenly scaled the fence – the same fence Blaxland had complained numerous times would not do to keep lunatics within – and made a dash down the immense slope to the bay. Finding the water, he dived in. He swam some way along the shore to get his bearings, stripped his clothes off and then began to swim across the bay towards the opposite shore. The attendants, always responsible for the relocation of escapees, followed in the steam-launch and collected him as he emerged from the water. Understandably exhausted, he had to be *carried* home – interestingly, not forced to walk. Once back in Ward Two he was 'well scrubbed and put into a warm bed, stimulants were administered and in an hour he was warm' again with 'no ill effects' following.

The next two years saw numerous occasions of seclusion for Parcelli who was 'inclined to make sudden attacks on people' and answered most questions with violence to both staff and fellow patients. Camisoles were used in the more extreme cases when he was violent. In late 1881 staff were forced to experiment with some different treatments for Parcelli, who was increasingly unmanageable in the small confines of Garryowen. Most of these remedies, to modern eyes, are remarkably questionable in terms of efficacy, but it is interesting to note the scientific interest of staff when such remedies appeared to take effect. Parcelli embarked upon a treatment which involved his restraint – this time his hands were disabled by leather muffs to stop him interfering with the treatment – and croton oil was rubbed on his head. This treatment was repeated several times over the New Year period of 1882 and his medical files were updated to read, 'After two rubbings he is somewhat brighter and better'. This procedure is virtually unheard of elsewhere and must have been based in the use of massage to release stress. Manning wrote in 1888 of the underutilization of remedial massage in the therapy of the insane.[6] Croton oil at this time tended rarely to be used topically – but rather as a laxative. Unsurprisingly to the modern reader, the perceived benefit did not last for long, and soon Parcelli was restrained with muffs daily and described as 'as untidy' and 'restless and mischievous as ever'. Blisters were tried next – the application of mustard powder or some other irritant to the head or neck to raise a swelling or blister. Along with administrating emetics to patients enduring an epileptic fit, and the inducement of vomiting, this was a type of 'heroic treatment' where health was sought through the restoration of the 'balance' in a body. This attitude was unusual in the nineteenth century, being regarded as somewhat archaic. Parcelli was subjected to this treatment to raise a blister on his neck in May 1882. No benefit was derived and the patient, unable to be calmed, was swapped with one of Gladesville's patients, Patrick Sighe. Callan Park acknowledged that the limited accommodation it could offer would not suit this particular Italian. His mischievousness made it impossible to properly care for him.

The Parcelli which Gladesville received was no better than when he had left. He was just as maniacal but now he spoke in Italian instead of English; added to this were a set of 'unascertained' delusions he was suspected of having recently developed. He refused to wear a hat or shoes and when supplied with them would throw them onto the roof. He was twenty-nine at this stage, but not particularly violent or unmanageable. For five months he was calm and controlled, until he relapsed and the staff at Gladesville were obliged to restrain him with muffs as had been done at Callan Park. Irritable and paranoid, Parcelli did not always get along with other patients. In 1884 he was involved in a fight with another patient and after a fall it became clear he had broken his leg. For a month and a half the leg was healing well, but the patient's 'mischievousness' made the attendants 'fasten him in bed' and later allocate a 'special Attendant [to] watch him day and night to prevent him leaving off his splints and bandages'. Clearly Parcelli outwitted this man sent to observe him, because a month later his leg bone was threatening to pierce his skin. He was put under chloroform to fix it, and less than a month later he was back in a general ward and being made to exercise the limb.

By September 1885 he was being forced to go out and work to aid in his rehabilitation, as per the ideals of Moral Therapy, despite the fact he was 'always trying to escape'. Between November 1885 and January 1889 Parcelli had numerous attempted and temporarily successful escapes. In November 1885 he escaped at 5pm but was 'retuned by two strangers at 8.15'. He tried again a month later, climbing a garden wall, but was found after forty-five minutes. A year later he re-enacted his Callan Park swimming marathon and swam across the Lane Cove River. He was returned three days later by the police. In May 1887 he escaped while working in one of the paddocks, and a year and a half later made the newspaper as the 'Italian Prince' after disappearing from a working party. Again, he was missing for three days. His last escape from Gladesville was at the beginning of 1889 when he vanished during a picnic but was swiftly returned by the police.

Four months later and rightly exhausted, Parcelli was described rather hopefully by staff as 'much more placid and does not attempt to escape'. By August 1891 he was much more 'trustworthy and tidy' but still not suitable for discharge. Manning sought independent advice about Parcelli and his treatment – ever keen to discharge patients from his hospital, particularly if he thought a patient might do better at home with his family. Dr V. Marano, an independent doctor from the Italian Consulate, whose offices where located in Hyde Park, visited Parcelli in March 1892 when Parcelli had begun to be quite idle and was still suffering from hallucinations of hearing. Writing to Dr Eric Sinclair, Gladesville's then medical superintendent and the man who would come to be New South Wales' second Inspector General of the Insane, Marano explained, 'I examined Parcelli this afternoon and found that his mental condition is still bad and that he would not be in a position to take care of himself if discharged from the asylum'. An indication of finality, the letter was signed by Sinclair and glued into Parcelli's *Medical Case Book* pages. Manning and Sinclair must have been disappointed for Parcelli. By 1893 the patient was openly talking to himself and imaginary people but had lost any interest in escaping. He had come to a junction in his life – one presumably accepting of his need for ongoing care. In 1894, then forty years old, it was noted that he was 'very ingenious at manufacturing false keys' but (and somewhat interestingly) 'does not try to escape himself'. He was regularly assisting the carpenter by this time.

Parcelli, as a chronic patient, was transferred to Kenmore in Goulburn in 1897. During World War II Kenmore was requisitioned by the Australian Armed forces and as a result the medical files of patients were destroyed. Details of Parcelli's improvement do not therefore exist, but there is no reason to think that he did not continue in his increase in health and calmness. His death in 1940, just as the hospital was being emptied of its insane patients, meant that he was buried in the grounds of Kenmore.

Parcelli and the other men who are discussed in this chapter are prime examples of the problem which faced New South Wales at the end of the nineteenth century in terms of foreign lunatics. The issue was two-fold: New South Wales' lunatic population was more and more made up of recent immigrants whose mental balance had been interrupted in the short time after their arrival. In addition, since New South Wales' asylums enjoyed an excellent reputation as to care and results, New South Wales became over time a dumping ground for the rest of the Commonwealth's insane population, with some clear lunatics going directly from port to Reception House immediately upon arrival in New South Wales. Understandably, this outraged New South Wales' tax payers, who were obliged to fund the treatment of such men and women. The issue lay mostly with the men and women who had been deliberately put aboard a ship to be delivered to the care of New South Wales – and often without any contribution to their upkeep. *Less* problematic were the foreigners who had *become* mad after having arrived sane – contemporary opinions seemed to take the view that this was fair enough, though they were not happy about it. It was those who had *arrived* as lunatics who were particularly the issue. Parliament regarded New South Wales' asylums as not 'equalled' and 'much less excelled, by those of other colonies, and as a consequence we were getting a large percentage of lunatics from the other colonies into our asylums'. The high level of care offered – including the safety and humanity with which patients were treated – made such conduct attractive to the families of the insane. The ministers went on: 'It was not fair to us, however, not only on account of the expense, but because it made it appear to the outside world that the proportion of lunatics to the whole population was larger than it really was'.[7]

Caring for these immigrants – whether they had been insane before arrival in New South Wales or not – was expensive, and the people of New South Wales bristled at supporting these economic vegetables. Part of the problem lay in the organisation of New South Wales' laws. In 1892, after numerous previous petitions by Manning during his time as Inspector General of the Insane, this was discussed in the New South Wales parliament:

> *There was a passenger on the Orient Company's steamer* Oroya *who was insane. When the vessel arrived in Melbourne the captain found he could not put the passenger on shore there unless he contributed to his support, but knowing that in this colony* [New South Wales] *we admitted people of the insane class, he brought him on here, where he was placed in the lunatic asylum. The Master-in-Lunacy desired that some payment should be made, the lunatic not having any means, and he wrote to the captain of the ship, and in reply the manager of the Orient Company sent a letter, from which the following is an extract, 'I should be glad to know under what statute or rule of law you propose claiming any payment from us in this case'.*[8]

Leaving insane passengers in New South Wales was therefore legal and easy for captains of ships, and happened regularly. Manning's *Annual Report* from 1881 shows his concern over the numbers of patients admitted directly from vessels. In 1881 Gladesville received twelve such patients, and Callan Park three.[9] In 1883 Manning pinpointed Great Britain, the neighbouring colonies and the South Sea Islands, as the biggest contributors to such immigrants.[10]

In 1886, out of a total of 3203 publicly-housed lunatics, only 856 were natives of New South Wales. 105 were from 'other colonies' in Australia, 940 from Britain, 947 from Ireland and 355 Frenchmen, Germans, Chinese, South Sea Islanders, African 'blacks' and a 'motley assemblage of wanderers from every part of the world'.[11] Whether these men and women were insane while travelling to New South Wales or became so once they arrived was increasingly irrelevant: New South Wales was shouldering the burden of these lunatics often for decades' worth of care.

The more common of the two situations was the latter: that the culture shock associated with New South Wales drove originally-well people mad. Manning cited isolation and sunstroke as the major contributors here, with unwary immigrants being thus struck down, due to a lack of preparation for the new conditions. Like Parcelli, who seems to have been well before his arrival in Queensland, many labourers in particular found illness a result of their new lives in Australia. Unsurprisingly, the conditions and stresses associated with activities such as goldmining meant that a proportion of Chinese goldminers found more than treasure in Australia. Such men, targets of racial discrimination, far from home and without family, struggling with the hot conditions, were sitting ducks for developing insanity.

Gold was first found in Australia by a shepherd in Bathurst in 1823. Three decades later, in 1851, Edward Hammond Hargraves made the first major discovery of gold at Ophir, near Bathurst.[12] The report of this find, published in the *Sydney Morning Herald* in May of the same year, conveyed the excitement of the discovery of gold:

> *GOLD, GOLD, GOLD – If anyone is incredulous to the fact of gold having been found in these districts, they need not be incredulous any longer. I have myself seen it, and I am perfectly satisfied there is no deception in the matter... Parties for the diggings are forming in every direction, and machines are being constructed for washing the soil, sand, &c. I hope that the Government will see the necessity*

of immediately strengthening the hands of the local authorities, by adding to the number of the constabulary or by forming a separate corps to preserve peace and order in these districts, for I assure you I much fear that crime and outrage of every description will soon be the order of the day. I hear there are upwards of two hundred persons on the gold ground, and the number is daily increasing.[13]

Thousands of miners flocked to Australia from both neighbouring colonies and the rest of the world, including China. By 1861 there were 11,000 Chinamen in New South Wales panning for gold; Victoria hosted 24,000. The 1860s witnessed a drop in the numbers of miners, and then a resurgence when gold was discovered in Cooktown in Queensland in the 1870s.

Anti-Chinese sentiment is clear from the sources of the time: in Victoria the government placed a tax on Chinese miners to enter the state and for their subsequent residence. The poll-tax was charged at a high £10 per person and was designed to discourage Chinese miners from arriving in the state but in reality merely forced the miners to adopt long cross-country routes to avoid the tax man. Anti-Chinese leagues were also rife, and sometimes turned violent. Thus were these Asian men inundated: largely unwelcome in Australia, plunged into an alien environment with harsh conditions in marked contrast to their home country, alone and separated from friends and family. The stresses of such a life were sometimes made clear, as in 1877 when there was a Chinese riot at Bathurst over a 'loose woman named Nutter'.[14] 'She had been insulted by members of the camp opposite to that in which she sat as queen, and her devoted admirers and slaves marched out to wreak vengeance upon the offenders'. During the fight blood 'flowed freely' with the 'Celestials ... in a great state of excitement'. This was a riot among two Chinese camps, an outlet for their frustrations. Many of the Chinese miners subsequently found gaol time the result of their actions; others were affected by depression and bouts of mania. Those who did found themselves transferred to Sydney, to Callan Park.

In Callan Park's early years three Chinese men[15] were admitted to Garryowen. They often spoke little English, making their state of mind sometimes hard to gauge. In addition, details of previous mental illness were impossible to be accessed, in order to assist with a clear diagnosis.

Twenty-six-year-old Chan Long arrived in Sydney onboard the vessel *Brisbane* in November 1875. His ship had docked briefly at Cooktown, where numerous miners alighted to find their fortunes in Queensland's earth; Long went on to New South Wales. Which mine he worked for, and which state it was in is unknown. Eventually, however, he arrived back in Sydney where, after exhibiting disturbing symptoms in public, he was picked up by the Water Police and delivered to Reception House. From there he was taken to Gladesville, the primary receiving asylum at the time. At Gladesville it became quickly evident that he could understand English but 'could not give a rational reply to even the simplest questions.' His dirty habits, both by day and night, demonstrated his inability to care for himself; he was erratic and suffered from frequent outbursts of rage. Adding an Oriental flavour to Garryowen, Long was transferred to Callan Park in the fourth group of twelve which arrived at the end of 1879. Described as a little better for his treatment at Gladesville, Long was also flagged as 'fanciful' and 'hypochondriacal' but 'by no means a troublesome patient'. Along with so many others, however, Long found his new environs in Balmain bewildering and immediately began numerous attempts to escape over the roofs of Garryowen. Staff responded with muffs – not personal violence – to restrain this agile man, though through 1880 he persisted in this behaviour whenever the restraint was withdrawn.

In 1881 Long's mental state began to calm, and his energy was replaced with a deep melancholia which meant that he often sat all day in the one position. A swollen leg, probably due to some escape attempt, did not help matters. In this time, Long's next of kin appear to have been notified of his treatment and residence at Callan Park, for in the following year a group of 'Chinamen' arrived to visit him. It was unusual for foreign patients to receive visitors, and this would have been an interesting break to the routine at Callan Park. To the staff's disappointment, however, these men had no English either, and merely conversed with Long in their own language before going away again. Frustratingly, they shed no light on the finer points of his condition. A year later Long was described rather thoughtlessly as 'dreadfully stout, his face looking not unlike that of a prize pig. No mental change'. Soon after, following an epileptic fit, he died – alone and unmourned – in early 1884.

One of Long's cultural comrades at Callan Park was Ah Fuun, and no doubt also a fellow victim of that flourishing sense of white European superiority. Also a Chinese miner, Fuun was not hampered by a lack of English. While mining in Bathurst, Fuun succumbed to the harsh Australian environment and suffered from an attack of sunstroke. Manning wrote extensively on sunstroke as a cause of insanity:

> *Practically sunstroke, as a cause of insanity, in England, is almost unknown. It is far from otherwise in this colony. Five per cent of the total number of cases are accredited to it, and I think with good reason ... Many slight attacks of illness assigned to other causes are I believe due to the effect of heat and glare on the cerebral circulation ... It is in the power of physicians to prevent such mischief by inculcating greater care in avoiding exposure, by insisting on a more rational head covering for the summer months than a black stove-pipe hat, and by pointing out that after an attack of sunstroke alcohol is an absolute poison, and cannot be taken with impunity in even small quantities. A person who has once suffered from sunstroke must be either a teetoller or a lunatic. There is, I believe, no middle standpoint.*[16]

Fuun, suffering dementia caused by this sunstroke, was arrested in 1877 and taken to Bathurst Gaol for the offence of 'unsound mind'. While there the gaolers were affirmed in their action: Fuun spent his time in his cell talking at length to an imaginary Chinese man. He destroyed his clothing and was sometimes so violent as to require restraint. In 1878, the forty-year-old, with no friends or family in Australia, arrived at Gladesville. Gladesville's doctors recorded not only sunstroke as the root of his problems: excessive use of that 'detestable habit of smoking opium'[17] was also suspected as a causal factor.

He oscillated between a silly, childish demeanour, an outrightly violent temperament and a manageable, helpful mindset. Overall though he was industrious, working in the gardens at Gladesville and in his ward. Sometime in 1878 he suffered a slight setback in his recovery, an 'attack' which left him tremulous and unsure.

In 1879 Fuun was transferred to Callan Park as a single patient outside the large and co-ordinated transfers. It is unclear why he was chosen for removal to the branch establishment at this time but it may have been as a translator for one of the other Chinese men there, Ah Chun. Ah Chun had been a sailor on a mail steamer. Found to be of unsound mind while aboard, the captain, unhindered by the kind of laws which restricted such dumping of lunatics in Victoria, abandoned Chun in Sydney in 1874. Forced to beg on the streets for some months, Chun arrived at Gladesville dirty, 'semi-idiotic' and having suffered a deep scalp wound. Treatment at Gladesville was successful and Chun, though still 'demented', was recorded as 'very useful'. Calm and manageable, he was among the first forty-four men to arrive at Callan Park. He was 'industrious' and well-behaved even when struck by another patient with a crockery pot. Finding companionship, he worked with Fuun in the laundry at Garryowen. In 1882 some friends arrived from China, and having the necessary money to send him back to China, he was discharged to their care.

Fuun, however, continued to work well at Callan Park after his transfer there, and even made the newspaper, *Freeman's Journal,* in July 1880:

> *It was here I had the honour of an introduction to a Chinaman named Ah Soon* [sic], *who, if his intellect was affected, by no means evinced it in either his manner or speech. He was a big, fine-looking copper-coloured fellow, and appeared to be on peaceable terms with the laundry-women, whom he was assisting in their various duties.*[18]

But before the article could be published Fuun was dead, falling during a post-dinner walk on the verandah at the front of Garryowen. Twenty hours later, the staff at the asylum conducted a *post mortem* on this patient:

> *The body was clean, fat ... All the internal organs were healthy. On opening the skull a small clot was found lying on and extending into the substance of the left hemisphere of the brain. The clot was about 1½ × 2 inches superficial measurement and was evidently the cause of his sudden death.*

The Coroner declined to hold an inquest.

In 1886 Manning[19] was explicit in his concern for patients such as these – while they lived. Aside from the fiscal issues in supporting them at the tax payers' expense, there was a further issue: patients who could not speak English presented a problem in the process of treatment. What were these men working towards? Manning did not know the answer: even if discharge could be granted, how could such patients have a fresh start in the colony if they could not function properly due to the language barrier? The care and treatment of lunatics was underpinned by a hope that they would one day be discharged – which is to say, that they could look after themselves and be regular contributors to New South Wales' society. But what could be done with those who would *never* be able to, because they were such recent immigrants in the colony?

One of these hopeless cases was the patient named Baroot.[20] Baroot was known in his notes only by his surname since his first name was unknown, due to his inability to speak English. Even on his 1882 death certificate it was unknown, and in the space where a Christian name would be recorded was the unhelpful descriptor 'Negro'. The staff at Callan Park, where he was immediately brought from Reception House in 1879, knew enough that he was married and had two children. He was also recorded as having been a coaler from Africa. Baroot is likely to have been Khumis Baroot who was listed as having departed from the African port of Muscat and arriving in Sydney in 1876 on the *Avoca*. During this sea journey he was violent and destructive enough to have been refused continued employment by his captain. He was supposed to have tried to jump overboard in a suicide attempt. Though the ship docked first at Melbourne, Baroot was purposefully abandoned in Sydney, just like Ah Chun.

It is unknown what he was doing between 1876 and his arrest in 1879 when he was thirty years old. At Callan Park he was described as 'very dull and stupid' besides suffering from melancholia. While at Garryowen he began to display a peculiar characteristic among those already there, many of whom had endured long stints as homeless: in stealing other patients' clothes. 'If allowed' he would put them on. Like many of his fellow patients, Baroot frequently wet himself at night, and it is highly likely that he would have been in one of the panelled rooms at Garryowen, near Parcelli. Like the Italian in 1881, Baroot was also restrained with muffs and had croton oil applied to his head in an attempt to treat his depression. In August 1882, the same month Parcelli was transferred back to Gladesville, Baroot, having been confined to bed with serious diarrhoea, died. As was the case with many 'foreign' and 'exotic' patients, he was naturally opened up soon after for his *post mortem* examination.

James Wilson Ellis, a 'tall old negro, with grey hair and whiskers', was the reverse of Baroot and would have been regarded as a much more hopeful case by Manning. Ellis was born in Jamaica, and had lived in Sydney, supporting his wife and child as a cook, for some years before he was committed to Callan Park. Despite his background, he spoke English well and had a strong family support system – for which it was worth attempting treatment to enable him to return to. Concerns over the point of attempting rehabilitation in regards to poor and non-English speakers did not apply to Ellis for this reason. Ellis was deeply disturbed by delusions related to grandeur and wealth. According to him, the Queen some time ago had made him a magistrate of £3000 per annum and that the people of Queensland had colluded to keep his rights from him. In his favour, however, was his imagined largesse in being a generous benefactor, a characteristic the majority of the insane added to their delusions. Further issues had arisen, Ellis said, when sailing from Cooktown while carrying a heavy cargo of gold: his ship had been looted by thieves. In reality, Ellis was a poorly-off sixty-eight-year-old who behaved himself well while at Callan Park. But he was never discharged back to the care of his wife:

Ellis died in 1882 of bronchitis and never left Callan Park.

The New South Wales public of the 1870s and 80s baulked at the cost of supporting these men – recent immigrants who had barely contributed to the society which would care for them and even bury them in death. These men were foreigners, dark and yellow skinned – visually and culturally 'other' to the 'white' and predominately British society of New South Wales. But not every inmate of Callan Park was out of step with the colony in this way. George Morton, a Londoner through and through, was a confirmed criminal and in 1872 had attempted the assassination of Queen Victoria. If Baroot and Parcelli were sometimes violent, Morton was downright dangerous, intent upon escape and deeply disturbed by Her Majesty.

7

GEORGE MORTON[1]

One day in 1872 almost seventeen-year-old Arthur O'Connor strolled by the Serpentine in Hyde Park in London, pondering the English monarchy. O'Connor was a highly-skilled clerk, able not only to read and write in a beautiful hand, but also possessed with literary ambition. He wrote poetry on his days off, and was imbibed with a keen sense, not altogether unfounded, of his poetic worth. On his slight shoulders he also carried a sense of grandeur, as the great nephew of Feargus O'Connor – the famous populist radical and Chartist leader who was immortalised in the popular song 'Lion of Freedom':[2]

> *The Lion of Freedom is come from his den;*
> *We'll rally around him, again and again;*
> *We'll crown him with laurel, our champion to be:*
> *O'Connor the patriot, for sweet Liberty!*

But gone were such days of fame and nation-wide gratitude: the current O'Connor generations lived in reduced circumstances, in a small house in Aldgate in London. George O'Connor, Arthur's father, collected tickets for a steamboat company. Arthur could not be satisfied with anonymity: his ambition was to gain notoriety for himself and claim back the fame which once came with the name O'Connor. His plan was to reach this by his writing – but he would gain it in quite another way entirely.

O'Connor was not an altogether well teenager. As a fourteen-year-old he had been hit by a cab in Chancery Lane and admitted to the London

Union Workhouse for treatment. He stayed there less than a week before being removed by his parents despite his head injury. Since that time he had had episodes of unpredictability, restlessness and pain in the head, with strange fancies occurring to him, which he sometimes acted upon. He was described at the time as 'a slight lad, with regular features, dark brown hair, long red hands and wrists protruding from his threadbare coat, with a wild expression of eye, a feverish flush in his thin cheeks'.[3] As O'Connor strolled through London in 1872, one of these sudden fancies occurred to him and he followed through.

The thought was one which would change the direction of his life: to attack Queen Victoria – but for what reason, not even O'Connor was really sure. One of his doctors, the famous[4] alienist Dr Thomas Harrington Tuke, described O'Connor's train of thought this day:

> *He told me that when walking by the Serpentine the idea suddenly struck him to shoot the Queen and thus release the 'Fenian Prisoners',*[5] *that he had no connection whatever with 'Fenianism', and had not thought of this before, that in the course of the day he reflected that the Prince of Wales would succeed, and that the Queen's death would be useless. He then determined to buy a pistol, to write out a free pardon for the* [Fenian] *prisoners, and an order for his own execution by shooting* [. T]*hat his plan was to hold a pistol, and to seize the Queen as she came out of the aisle of St Paul's Cathedral, and to hold a pistol to her head and while all around were paralysed with horror to order pen and ink to be brought and to compel her Majesty to sign the pardon. I argued with him upon this as to the frightful scene he would have made in the Cathedral* [. H]*is answer was he did not care* [,] *that he looked on the Queen as a political subject, and not as a woman only, and he was determined to carry out his purpose. He said it was perfectly justifiable and would most certainly have succeeded,* [despite the fact] *that at the age of fifteen he had been stunned by a blow on the head, that he had suffered from ill-health ever since ...* [6]

In actual fact O'Connor did not attack Victoria at St Paul's, since he had been unable to get close enough. Instead, he had been forced to wait until she arrived at the palace. John Brown, the personal attendant of the Queen, described the actual attack initiated by O'Connor:

> *Her Majesty went out for a drive in an open carriage. Her Majesty sat on the right of the carriage, and Lady Churchill* [her lady in waiting] *on the left. Opposite to the Queen was Prince Arthur. I was riding in the rumble behind. There were two equerries riding on either side of the carriage, and behind were two grooms. When the carriage stopped for the purpose of the Queen alighting, Lady Churchill was on the side nearest to the entrance. I got down to open the carriage door and saw the boy* [O'Connor] *coming up between the two equerries. He got up to within a yard of the carriage door. I thought there was something wrong, and shifted him back; Lord Charles Fitzroy also pushed him back, thinking he was one of the gardeners. He then rushed round to the Queen's side of the carriage. I followed him as fast as I could. When I got around he had just raised his hand to the top of the carriage. I just caught hold of him by the neck and one arm, and he dropped a pistol from his right hand, his left being then on the carriage. One of the equerries, General Harding, picked up the pistol, I keeping hold of the boy, I kept hold of him till a lot of people came running up with a policeman, and then I thought it time to give him up. The Queen was still in the carriage.*[7]

The Queen was astonished. O'Connor, a boy with no particular skills in weaponry or agility, had almost reached her carriage: a carriage which held herself and her two sons, Princes Arthur and Leopold. O'Connor was hauled off for questioning. But it was quickly clear that perhaps O'Connor was not of completely sound mind.

It was fast established by police that he had not intended to actually hurt Victoria. For one, the pistol was both unloaded and incapable of actually firing.[8] Secondly, O'Connor seemed to think that by merely approaching the Queen he should have been executed, and that this was actually his aim since he 'desired to have [his] life taken by the Law, my object was to have my life taken away'.[9] Indeed, had this fact been lost on Victoria in the chaos of having a pistol held to her head, at the end of the document he had drafted containing the instructions for the release of the Fenian prisoners, a postscript read:

> *Witnessed by – Whereas a person named Arthur O'Connor, residing at 4, Church – row, Houndsditch, in the City of London, having committed an outrage against my Royal person, has surrendered himself into my hands, he, the said Arthur O'Connor, being perfectly willing to suffer for such offence: Now, I, the said Victoria, Queen of Great Britain and Ireland, do solemnly pledge my Royal word to the effect that if the said Arthur O'Connor be found guilty of death by my judges, after a just and fair trial, he (the said Arthur O'Connor) shall not be strangulated like a common felon; but shall receive a death which is due to him as a Christian, a Republican, and as one who has never harmed a human being – that is to say he shall be shot, and after death his body shall be delivered to his friends to be buried wheresoever they may choose.*[10]

The police were faced with a prisoner of unsound mind: to the public observer it appeared that O'Connor had approached the Queen with a view to assassination. To the police, it seemed that O'Connor's reasons for intimidating the Queen were without logic or clear motive; that he had wished to die and had chosen this unusual – and extremely public – method to achieve his aim. He had no link to Fenianism, and appeared to be only an unhappy clerk with mild delusions. In addition, he had not actually even touched the Queen.

O'Connor made his first public court appearance at Bow Street in 1872. The court was described as being 'thronged with people' including the offended Princes who had witnessed the outrage.[11] The teenage O'Connor – alternately called 'the boy' and 'the prisoner' by the officials – was described as 'nonchalant', holding 'himself with an air of the utmost indifference to the charge against him, although there was nothing in his bearing to indicate bravado' and he appeared undefended in the court. The charge against him was only that he had 'presented a pistol to the Queen, with the intention to alarm her majesty',[12] and having virtually nothing to say for himself after witness testimony, he was committed for trial in the Central Criminal Court later the same month.

The fame which O'Connor had craved, he was now receiving, but not in the domain in which he had intended. On the day of his trial he was brought up with a bigamist, a killer, a burglar, several debtors, a forger and a church breaker. Undoubtedly the headline in such a line up, O'Connor's sense of his own grandeur and status must still have been taken aback.

At the start of his trial, O'Connor raised eyebrows when he stated his intention to plead *guilty*. His lawyer, Mr Hume Williams, being absent at that moment, was rather surprised to learn what his client had done. Upon his return, Williams asked that this plea might be re-entered and he asked permission to give evidence of O'Connor's lack of sanity. A jury having been empanelled, the question of O'Connor's possible insanity was tried, with O'Connor's parents and doctor examined.[13] Under cross-examination, O'Connor's father was forced to admit that in his own heart he did not believe his son was insane, but that 'it was a question for the medical man, not him, to decide'.[14] His mother agreed, keen to avoid the taint of insanity over her family. Dr Tuke, O'Connor's doctor, had been asked by O'Connor's father to visit his son while at Newgate. The two men knew each other from the treatment of Feargus O'Connor, where the doctor's knowledge had impressed George O'Connor; now Tuke gave evidence of Arthur O'Connor's insanity. The doctor was verbally attacked in court over this opinion: the Attorney General cross-examined him extensively, suggesting that Tuke had some personal motive for involvement in O'Connor's trial. Unbelievably, Arthur was found by the jury to be sane and therefore guilty of the attack on Her Majesty. Arthur O'Connor, who had wished only to die that day, was sentenced to one year's hard labour and 'to be once whipped, twenty strokes with a birch rod'.[15]

Guilty, the criminal O'Connor was moved from Newgate to the Middlesex House of Correction at Clerkenwell in April 1872 to serve his sentence. It did not take long for the reality of his sentence to sink in: O'Connor was a common felon, entirely lacking glory and fame. In November the same year, O'Connor wrote a petition[16] to the Secretary of State, asking for a more lenient punishment. He argued that he had acted alone and had never intended to kill the Queen. He reminded the Secretary that he had no connection with the much-maligned Fenians and acknowledged that 'I was not in full possession of my mental faculties [when I approached the Queen]. I was not mad, nor was I perfectly sensible'. He laid the blame for his actions at the doorstep of his ill health and explained that he was filled with 'continual remorse' for the shock he had caused Her Majesty. Anxiously, he asked for the flogging to be removed from his sentence – interestingly, this was a repetition of the same fear of suffering which had caused him to ask the Queen to have him shot rather than hanged – but instead reasoned that it 'would subject me to intolerable shame and lifelong reproach'. Most significant however was his discussion of the idea of his removal ('at perfect liberty and free from police suspicion') overseas to reduce the stress caused to the Queen and her minders once his release from prison had been effected. It is unclear if this 'removal' – an early release from prison – was O'Connor's idea or the government's – but whoever's it was, it quickly became the government's favourite solution to the O'Connor problem.

Thus began the negotiation between the British government and felon Arthur O'Connor as to where the latter would go to relive the stress on Her Majesty and her staff. The confidence and stubbornness of O'Connor spoke to his highly-inflated sense of self-worth and power in this situation. In the numerous letters exchanged between himself and the Secretary of State he corresponded with a grandeur hard to equate with an inmate at Clerkenwell. He depicts himself as a hyper-sensitive gentleman, one with reasonable reservations about the plan offered to assist him in avoiding much of his punishment. The nonchalance exhibited at Bow Street was fully realised here again: he writes as though the favour was his to give, rather than he being the beneficiary.

In December 1872, a few weeks into the negotiations, he declared that he would be happy to assist her Majesty in his removal, but that a *permanent* exile from England would be impossible:

> *For myself I am willing to go to the place mentioned, but the remaining there, during Her Majesty's life, without once returning to see those who naturally are dear to me is a most painful and trying proposition. At present Her Majesty as far as I know is in perfect health and will I sincerely hope continue so. Consequently there is no reason to suppose otherwise then that she will live a number of years yet, twenty or perhaps thirty. Much longer than I myself judging from my present debility and the generally fatal prospects of consumption can expect to live.*
>
> *Leaving out this however; during such a term, the lives of members of my family might terminate.* [One is] ... *already past sixty and who was when I last saw her far from well. Whatever my friends in their desire to relieve my present misery may consent to; I can never agree to a condition which would condemn me to almost perpetual exile; and which would be rendered a living death by the knowledge that the dearest of my relations might pass from this life while I thousands of miles away could only cry out against that which withheld me from them at such a moment and wonder at the attributes of that Providence which has sent me into the world and which, from my cradle has not allowed me a single year's relief from suffering and has ended by adding to it the miseries and shame of animal confinement. If Sir the above condition were modified; I at least should have no further objection to the proposal, being by this time weary of an existence so useless and contemptible and deserving only death if further life will bring no alteration.*[17]

Taking these provisions as a given, he quickly moved on to the fine details he expected to be managed by the government on his behalf:

I am doubtful what employment would suit me best. Certainly nothing at all sedentary or confined. It is that kind of work which has more than anything else assisted me in my downward prospects. My disposition is naturally opposed to it. Rather than sit at the desk for a single hour I would labour a whole week in a clearing. And if the choice of employment were offered me I should gladly choose that requiring continual activity and exertion in the open air for altho' pressed down at present by languor and weakness; which makes activity of mind or body impossible I am certain that a few weeks passed in pure bracing air would restore both. Looking upon every event and especially this that occurs to me as directed by the finger of God, I feel instinctively that this is the turning point of my life. It appears no doubt somewhat strange to look to Providence for the explanation of this occurrence. The practical man would smile at such an assertion; the Christian doubt; and the Physician solve the whole by muttering lunacy or some such influence. But the ways of God are not the ways of man. Was there anything opposed (I speak in the moral sense) to his nature in the idea I would not hold such a belief for a moment. But I know the contrary, I know that however wild and absurd; there was no harm whatever meant nor no dishonesty employed in its execution; and when I reflect upon the consequences which have resulted from it to myself of the change from a furious atheist cursing nature for my existence; to a plain believer in the Providence Almighty and hereafter of God – from a misanthropic, hypochondriac; to a hopeful cheerful convalescent; from a wild thoughtless youth; to a sober reflecting man; it is not suspicion but conviction which fills my mind, such conviction rendering me proof against all the fears of the future and giving me hope, tranquillity, confidence and strength. Apologising for the length of this letter.

I have the honour to remain Sir
Yours most obed and respectfully
Arthur O'Connor[18]

The government was swift and blunt in its reply: it grappled with O'Connor's grandeur and control, crushing these, and managed to put him in his place. O'Connor baulked at this and hurriedly replied with a response cool and stubborn but, this time, a little rattled:

> *Sir,*
> *I cannot accept a pardon that has any conditions whatever attached to it. I have been so long deprived of liberty that it is now the only thing to which I look forward to and I should hereafter be perfectly miserable were I to know that my free will and inclination were in the slightest degree confined. From what has occurred, I conclude that the Home Office believes me to be possessed of a Royal mania or something of the sort and that for H Majesty's safety and peace of mind they desire me to leave the country. I can understand this and I am quite willing to go abroad not as a Government Prisoner as it were but as an independent and unrestrained individual paying for my passage from my own means and going to whatever part of the country my inclination leads me and returning when I wish to do so.*
>
> *There was no supervision included in my sentence and it appears to me that none could be exercised upon me unless I was to be tried again and a new sentence with supervision included passed upon me.*
>
> *If I am flogged it will be not an act of justice but of cruelty, I was not in a responsible state when that act was committed and if the Law had handed me over to the Physician instead of the Jailer justice and humanity would have been both satisfied. Altho' Sir this is my decision I give it firmly believing that no decision of mine or of anyone else can prevent me from entering upon any other sphere than that prepared for me by the destiny of God.*[19]

These letters were carried via the head of Middlesex Correctional House, and in late 1872, he advised the Secretary of State that even though the

O'Connors visited their son and made clear that they desired him to serve his sentence rather than going abroad, he had sent O'Connor 'paper to write the enclosed, merely hinting that if he [O'Connor] did not accept the conditions he might have to suffer the whole sentence, and remain a marked man in this country'.[20] This plan worked: O'Connor accepted the government's offer. He would be sent to Australia, provided with a position which suited his skill set, and be watched over by the Inspector General of Police in New South Wales. O'Connor was still not satisfied with this, writing in February 1873, 'What have I to do with police now? Am I not a free independent person and who but incorrigible rogues have anything to do with them [police]. No honest man would unless he wished it and I am such and I do not wish it'.[21] But he accepted nonetheless and his father, purchasing for his son the ticket and a new outfit (at a cost of 45 guineas and £20), had the audacity to send the bill to the government,[22] along with a request a month later for £10 to cover the expenses he had been put to throughout the trial and incarceration of his son.[23]

By June 1873, O'Connor was officially New South Wales' problem and not England's. He had been released early from his hard labour, and had had his flogging entirely cancelled. England breathed a sigh of relief and New South Wales prepared to manage the self-proclaimed literary genius. As soon as O'Connor arrived, Hercules Robinson, governor of New South Wales, wrote to Lord Kimberley in England. Robinson reported that O'Connor had arrived safely and followed the instructions given to him that he should immediately report to Robinson's private secretary. O'Connor was put in contact with the colonial secretary and the superintendent of police who were to 'look after [O'Connor]'.[24] Robinson went on:

> *Inquiries were made with the object of providing him employment and he has now taken a situation for six months with a butcher named Geary at Morpeth, a farm on the Hunter River, where he is to receive ten shillings a week with board and lodging, and where his duties, I am informed, will be to keep the Shop*[']*s Book, and* [illegible] *out for orders.*[25] *He left for Morpeth on the 11th instant*

> *... He confesses himself, however, much disappointed with the place as not offering a field for the exercise of the literary talents which he thinks he possesses.*[26]

Robinson also enclosed with his own correspondence a letter written by O'Connor which the latter intended to be forwarded to the Queen. The letter never made it, but was instead added to the expanding Home Office file with O'Connor's name on it in England. There were growing indications that O'Connor was not as well as was assumed. Dr Tuke had called him insane upon their first meeting, and continued to label him so, and now Robinson must have wondered what exactly he had been burdened with by the mother country.

> *June 11 1873*
> *To Victoria, Queen of Great Britain and Ireland*
> *Most Gracious Madam,*
>
> *Being told previous to my leaving London, that on my arrival I was to write to your Majesty, I now obey –*
>
> *I left London on the 12th of February and arrived in Sydney on the 20th of May.*
>
> *The passage was a most miserable one to me from the fact of my bad health, and there being no other Cabin Passengers, but myself – consequently when I had read all the books I brought with me I had no way of amusing myself but by writing and I dared not do much of that, as the mental strain injured me – I could have passed some pleasant hours with the sailors, in their cabin, but for the Captain, who would not allow me to go there. He treated me most insultingly all through the voyage, without my giving him any provocation so to do.*
>
> *When we were first out of sight of land I was much struck and pleased with the sublimity of the boundless ocean, as I had never been to sea before and everything was new to me. We had fine weather, through the Channel but on the 24th of the same month,*

a heavy gale set in, and lasted several days. We were not damaged by it. As this was my first sea experience, I suffered much from sea sickness but bore it contentedly, knowing it is generally productive of good.

My great expectation were the Tropics. Here the warm weather, so balmy, the refreshing breezes, the gorgeously beautiful sunsets, the superb moonlights, and the strange fish all pleased me greatly.

My whole life had been passed in London. I had never before experienced Nature's garden nor even her simpler influence, though I used to pant for it, and this sudden entry into her most sublime, and beautiful dominion almost overpowered me.

The sunny day[s], *were all great joys to me, stupefied as I was, by London smoke and gloom.*

There is something indescribably beautiful and affecting in a true summer's day.

An odour, a peace, a sense of etherial loveliness in which the soul [illegible], *it mingles ineffably with the thoughts, speaking to them in a voice, which we cannot define, but which is certain and sympathetic, raising within us a boundless yearning for closer union more lasting and more comprehensible. It is part of the pure essence of God foreshadowing the entry of man, into its perfection.*

We left the tropics early in April. On passing the Cape of Good Hope the weather was very different, being winter there and to the end of the voyage. For a whole month we laboured day, and night, mid of fearful seas, pursued continually by storms and hurricanes. The sight of the raging sea with its mountainous waves, thundering over and around the ship, as if they would bury her every moment, was an extraordinary one to me, so unused to it, and forced me on my knees, in adoration of the immensity and might of God.

The ship was much damaged by the heavy seas. She leaked dangerously and had to be pumped out continually. In such a ship, with a bullying Captain possessing neither courtesy, nor kindness, without a soul to speak to, with[out] *profit or pleasure, having nothing to read nor to do, weak, listless, and half stupefied at time I had but one solace, my pen – it being then that I wrote the accompanying letter. It is my vindication, and if your Majesty so pleases, I could almost desire it to be published. Its style, that of verse, comes most natural, and easy to me – God is good – He has afflicted me much, but in return, he has given me a mind, which supplies all wants, which is my world, which is full of riches a thousand times dearer to me than gold or diamonds –– Whose fathers are Homer and Milton and all the Sons of Song.*

On 14th of May came the welcome cry of 'land ho!' We were now in the smooth waters and the land was Cape Otway [in the state of Victoria, Australia].

After so much rough weather and tossing about, it was indeed pleasant, to sail smoothly past beautiful scenery and towns, and villages. Everything was just like home. The harbour of Sydney is grand – I do not like the town, it is so dull and small, compared to London. The people, the climate, and the scenery I like very much. The people especially I admire. They have none of that proud reserve and distrust that is so strong in England but are homely, kindly and generous. I was treated most kindly, by the Government Gentleman to whom I had letters. I have changed my name, to George Morton, as the people being very loyal, I might suffer some annoyance were I to be known. In the room in which I write, there is a fine painting of Your Majesty, set in a frame exquisitely carved, by one of the young ladies of the house. No situation being offered me I obtained one myself up the Country at Morpeth, a days journey from Sydney by steamer.

It is a poor one, but I took it, because I could not bear being dependant so much on and living by, others.

The business, a Butchers, is distasteful to me owing I suppose to my poetic disposition.

I shall be a sort of general clerk. The wages are poor, which of course I must expect, as I shall have to learn a great deal.

I have not the slightest intention of settling out here – I shall remain only till my health is restored, then return some and strive for literary eminence.

I have no right to be away from home. I am the second son. My elder brother, possessed of great and powerful talents, forsook a fine prospect and inlisted like a common navvy. He will I have no doubt excel there, as he excelled everywhere else, possessing as he does a powerful mind and education.

My duty, the sacred duty of my life, is to fill his void, and attend to the comfort and happiness of those, who so long attended to me.

It is in literature that I shall get on – I cannot bear business, I am not fitted for it. I would rather be an independent writer, living in a garett, most poorly, than a business man worth £500 a year.

There is no mind so peculiar, so distinct and so strong in its yearning, as a poet's. It stands alone, and lives in a glorious solitude, apart from the world, and to its music, the sounds of trade, are death. It is a heavenly blossom, that would spring up into glory, in a desert, but which would die despairingly amidst the horrors of the Counting House.

Oh how I long to escape the practical demon that ties me to the desk and maddens me. How I long for the solitude, and peace, of the woods in whose depths, deep, deep, in the heart of Nature with the dazzling forms of my fathers ever around me, breathing music I would find pure, continual and perfect joy and peace – wanting nothing beyond my thoughts.

There is one prize [the position of Poet Laureate] *towards which I am ever looking – none but a poet can obtain it, and as yet I think, no Irish poet has held it. Passionately Irish myself, this honor I will bring upon Ireland, poor Ireland, if the highest limit of human shining can obtain success. It comes from the throne, and is now held by a writer yet 'not one of the grand old masters'. He is not immortal. I beseech Your Majesty to read the accompanying letter. It will shew that if I sinned, I suffered also, and deserved more, far more pity than punishment.*

I have written this, as I was told to write naturally, and as though it were to my mother.

God bless and keep Your Majesty

Arthur O'Connor.[27]

O'Connor was George Morton now. He went off to Geary's butcher shop in Morpeth in the Hunter Valley to work. But such a job was beneath George Morton: he was a poet, not a meat curer, and Morpeth not exactly a humming centre where one might achieve literary fame. Mrs Geary in particular seems a frightening female figure: in 1884[28] while coming to the aid of two victims of assault in Morpeth she was accosted by one of the villains. She promptly knocked down her attacker with one swift hit, unaided. These were uncultured people in Morton's eyes: rough and without subtlety or knowledge of good literature. In a very short time Morton found himself bored of Morpeth and he gave his notice, and simply returned to Sydney expecting to be found a new job.[29] But this would take time – and was a difficult prospect since employment required disclosure of one's real name, not an alias, and the government feared the public unmasking of Morton. The Inspector General of Police was obliged to support Morton with public money in the interim.[30]

Henry Parkes was drafted in to assist in the finding of new employment for Morton – this time in Sydney, so that a closer eye could be kept on him, and since Sydney, being a big city, was more suited to his desire for literary eminence. Parkes was successful – he called in a favour from Mr J. C. Brown, who had his own solicitors' firm in Sydney. Brown had 'kindly interested himself in Morton's case',[31] and having been offered the position of colonial treasurer previously, Parkes decided Brown could be trusted to keep Morton's real identity secret. Brown offered Morton the job of copying clerk in his leading Sydney firm.[32] Robinson wrote happily to Lord Kimberley explaining this change in Morton's circumstances, and with the hope that Morton would 'appreciate' this kind offer and make the most of it.

But a month passed and Morton, characteristically, was not satisfied. Robinson was forced to write to Lord Kimberley again:

> *... George Morton called on my Private Secretary a few days since, and by his own account he seems to be well satisfied with his employment in Mr Brown's office. He is, however, only seeking at present the annual salary of fifteen shillings a week, an amount which is sufficient and indeed liberal in the case of young men who have board and lodging found for them by their parents, but the sum is insufficient to enable Morton to live respectably. He is accordingly for the present receiving from the Police Department a supplementary allowance of £1 a week, an expenditure of which I trust your Lordship will approve.*[33]

Perhaps Morton was tired of Sydney and its lack of literary culture, perhaps repulsed by the connection he was forced to maintain with the police in supplementing his income, when he thought he should be free. Whatever the cause, Morton decided to leave Australia in April 1874, after having been in New South Wales for less than a year. He did Robinson the courtesy of warning his private secretary of his intentions, but showed no other gratitude for what had been done for him. There was no legal basis for keeping him in Sydney or indeed out of England. Certainly he had had his sentence torn up by the English government in exchange for his leaving Britain, but there was no law to say he could not return. Robinson was painfully aware of this, but unable to stop him. He expressed surprise at Morton's decision to leave, writing to Mr Robert Meade at the Colonial Office that 'he was doing well [at Brown's office] and would have got on – however he was quite determined to go'.[34] Brown even tried to dissuade Morton from leaving, offering to raise his weekly salary from 15s to 25s.[35] Suddenly Morton's complaints about his salary at Brown's were made embarrassingly transparent:

> *It would seem that this young man has from the first been dissatisfied and he has probably been following out a design for* [illegible] *part to leave the colony; for although representing to my Private Secretary from time to time that his allowance was insufficient for this maintenance he has in some way become possessed of £16 which sum it appears he disbursed for his passage to England.*[36]

Robinson was unsure how to proceed: Parkes and the Inspector General of Police were absent from Sydney when Morton made his announcement, and so he had no one with whom to confer who was also aware of Morton's true identity.[37] Robinson considered asking the master of the ship Morton was to sail in to decline his passage but feared that if he did this, he would be unable to give details to England via which they could track Morton's journey and meet him upon his arrival.[38] Robinson, apparently trying to comfort Lord Kimberley at this unsettling turn of events, and unable to take any action to stop Morton, added in one of his many letters (which were accompanied by harried telegraphs) that 'Both Mr Brown and Mr Parkes have been favourably impressed with his demeanour and intelligence; and he informed Mr Brown when taking his leave that there was no need for the Authorities in England to feel uneasy about his return as he would never again give any trouble or annoyance'.[39]

Though Morton was under surveillance from his first step on home soil he was largely left alone. But he was not well: his symptoms were retuning, and more virulent than before. He wrote several letters to Dr Tuke, some of them acknowledging that it was on an 'impulse' that had he left Australia, the same type of impulse which had led him to attack the Queen. Other letters detailed his tendency to suicide and other symptoms. In one extensive memorandum and in a fit of self-examination he listed his ever-changing ailments:

> *Physical symptoms – back like ice – wind after eating – want of ability to swallow food – sickening in stomach – blood spitting at times – sexual excitement and continual nocturnal emissions. In*

cold weather one moment deadly chilled the next hot as fire – pains in the head – completely stupefied by cold weather – mental – want of rest – thought continually revolving upon religion – visions at night of angels hurling men precipices to die forever because they had not given up all they loved to go and sell Bibles to the unconverted – sense that unless I gave up the drama, witty and happy society, and the world generally I should be everlastingly damned – in a word, one unceasing mania concerning Jesus Christ the intellect warring with the mania yet unable to crush it – sense of utter want of constitution and energy, a feeling as if I were half dead – Naturally I am poetical – loving the Dramatic writers and poets of nature, and desirous of imitating them – at one time of my life that is before I became utterly debilitated and subject to the above symptoms, I was quite insusceptible to the present mania, which leaves me no rest day or night. Naturally I am devoured by energy, running in my walk, and in everything else, but when stupefied by dyspepsia scarcely able to drag a foot – of late my brain agony has been terribly increased. I awoke the other night raging to commit suicide the idea presented itself as a very delightful one, but just as I was about to leap from my bed, I recovered my senses and fell back trembling, and utterly horrified. Since then my feelings have risen to absolute madness continually, and I know I think so at least, that unless I recover from my bodily disease sooner or later delirium will come upon me.

My home is very wretched, it is in fact a hell to me.[40]

It was a long time coming, but in April 1875 Morton was finally arrested for being a 'person of unsound mind' after acting suspiciously at St James' Park, very close to the site of his attack on the Queen. On the afternoon in question, Detective Police Sergeant Daniel Davey and Sergeant Lansdowne were walking the park and at two o'clock saw Morton there. They saw nothing suspicious originally in Morton's behaviour until the Guards' Band marched into view. They watched Morton become suddenly and unnaturally excited, pushing to the front of the crowd in a great ecstasy. After the band moved on he became suddenly quiet again and then quickly vanished from sight. They managed to find him however and he was followed and arrested, telling the policemen: 'I expected I should see some of you, and that some of you would follow me'.[41] Morton was taken to Scotland Yard, where he was observed. He did not sleep, complained of wanting to 'destroy himself' and took pleasure only in his 'reading, writing and study'.[42]

The police wanted Morton committed. They called in Dr Tuke to give evidence as to Morton's insanity. Having been of the opinion that Morton was insane at his trial, and having recently received a letter from him, Tuke was not surprised to see Morton still unwell; indeed, worse than he had been. In his testimony Tuke stated that several of the O'Connor family members had been found insane over the years and Morton was clearly suffering from the same hereditary madness. Tuke saw a man in the same disarray as he had been in Newgate when they had first met. He declared at Scotland Yard:

> *I then found him unnaturally excited, his pulse was very fast, his eyes glistening, with much the same appearance of head and brain irritations as I have seen him in Newgate. He talked excitedly, he told Dr Tweedie and myself that he had an impulse towards suicide the week before, that he was sure he should be a 'grand person' some day, that he had made an offer to write all the Dramatic literary work in a magazine, and could do that in two night's work. He talked other exalted ideas on the same subject, the fact of his being found in the very same place where he had formerly held a pistol to the Queen's forehead, his very depressed and debilitated condition and his impulse to suicide the week before led me to the impression that his mind had again become unsound, and that until his health was restored he would always be liable to impulse, which might lead to inquiry to himself and distress and alarm, if not hurt, to the Queen.*

Tuke was direct in his evidence, ending with, 'I think he requires medical care and attention, and that his mind is not strong, on account of his health'.[43]

Like in New South Wales, two doctors' opinions were needed to install anyone in one of England's asylums. The second doctor was another who had visited Morton at Newgate during his trial, Alexander Tweedie. At the time of the trial Dr Tweedie had been convinced that Morton was of sound mind and refuted Tuke's assertion that Morton was in need of medical help. Called upon now, however, he said that Morton's insanity was clear and that Morton could not 'be considered responsible for his actions'. Tweedie even thought it 'very doubtful if he [could] recover his strength of mind'. Writing to Tuke, Tweedie warned of the consequences if Morton was not committed:

> *A further element in his mental condition should not be overlooked – the insanity of his late grand uncle Feargus O'Connor and other branches of his family. You may remember that I was summoned to attend this gentleman professionally when he committed a violent and unprovoked assault in the House of Commons on one of its members, and it is remarkable that he too for many months previously had exhibited similar strange fancies as his grand nephew Arthur O'Connor. You are aware that Fergus* [sic] *O'Connor was soon afterwards found to be of unsound mind after a judicial enquiry before Mr Barlow one of the Masters in Chancery – Benevolence.*[44]

George O'Connor agreed now, desiring that his son be treated by medical professionals particularly because of his suicidal tendencies. For his part, Morton insisted that he had not been acting strangely but 'I was thinking what a wonderful calm reigned in London, and that it was owing to the perfection of the Government'.[45] This didn't quite cut it for Tuke and Tweedie, who signed Morton's blue Lunacy Warrant, and he was taken to Hanwell Asylum in London.[46] Hanwell was a pioneering state institution which by O'Connor's time had entirely done away with any kind of restraint, and was a place where the patients spent much of the day outside, working.

Under the care of staff at Hanwell Morton improved. Given time to write, along with support, he recovered, and after a year and a half he was discharged as cured. He was released back into London and he returned to Aldgate to his family. But the O'Connors were not a happy, flourishing species: his father having died by this time, Morton found that he was now the breadwinner of his family and took up work again as a clerk. His mother was by this stage a drunk and offered little support to her fragile son, who craved a supportive home environment almost as much as literary fame. Morton struggled in this situation, suffering 'ill health' and hardly living in the best place for mental recuperation. He could not write and was distracted by his own weakening health. He decided to contact the British government, that fixer of all of his problems. No doubt to their extreme relief, he told them he wanted to leave his dreary life in London and to return to Sydney.[47] They quickly assented, and Morton set sail in early January 1881, never to return to England. Though Augustus Loftus was the New South Wales governor now, the procedure was the same: Parkes would arrange employment for Morton and the Inspector General of Police would provide a weekly allowance until a job was found, and then watch his movements.[48]

Sydney was ready: Parkes had prevailed upon Mr Brown to offer Morton another job and Mr Fosbery, the head of police, was ready to receive him. But Morton was still not completely well, and unable to conduct himself in the manner required. Perhaps Morton was still imbibed with the sense that he was somewhat above the law, as his past interactions with authority had taught him. Having only just arrived in the colony, free of familial duties, he was arrested for drunkenness. He was swiftly arrested and locked up – as anyone would have been. Even with his unusual background, Morton was not a special case and this was not a 'gotcha' moment for which the British and New South Wales governments might have congratulated themselves. Morton had transgressed the laws of New South Wales, and he was taken to court for it. But even at court Morton was still unable to control himself. Though sober, in the Police Court he was unaccountably violent and even injured a policeman in a struggle.[49] Loftus wrote to Lord Kimberley, clearly unimpressed at what he had been lumbered with: 'Mr Fosbery considers that he is insane, and a very dangerous character, and seems to entertain no doubt that he will have to be confined in a Lunatic Asylum'[50] since he was a danger to both himself and the public. Parkes agreed, saying that '"on his first visit he was a thoughtless youth, he has now become an unmitigated ruffian"' and wondered aloud why Morton had been given passage to New South Wales, rather than being confined in England.[51]

Morton was labelled as dangerous and could not be let free to go to his job with Brown as had been the plan. Instead, Morton was transferred from the Water Police Office, where he had been held, to Reception House, on 11 July 1881. Such a stay must have echoed Hanwell like nothing else for Morton and made it clear to him that he had relapsed. He stayed there for two days before being transferred on 13 July to Callan Park under the name of Morton. In Manning's *Register*[52] of all patients in New South Wales he was recorded as 'Morton or O'Connor, George' and in very light pencil was added 'fired at Queen Victoria'. Initially Manning was hopeful of his fast recovery: Morton was not expected to be a long term patient, with Manning writing to Fosbery in September 1881 to say that improvement had been made, but a little more care was needed before Morton might be discharged.[53] In this interchange of letters, copies of which were added to Morton's Home Office file in England, Manning and Fosbery were open and frank. Even Morton, one of the most inconvenient men in the Commonwealth, was not to be just thrown into Callan Park with the key thrown away. Even a would-be assassin of Her Majesty was not to be treated with any less dignity than a normal patient of Callan Park. Manning would not allow Callan Park to act as a holding pen or gaol, wielded as a punishment for England's criminals.

At Callan Park the staff entered Morton into their books. He was only twenty-five, and it was decided that his melancholia was caused by a combination of masturbation and syphilis – the disease which had claimed Feargus O'Connor's reputation and wits – the evidence being the scars of buboes on Morton's body. Information concerning his previous attacks was given – though not the subject of his initial delusions – and no family details were provided. He was described as being 'normal in expression' with 'good features' and that he ascribed 'all his troubles to faults of temperament'. Morton was still fearful of his wellbeing despite being in good bodily health. In alignment with Manning's ideas, and in sympathy with what had occurred at Hanwell, initially Morton was described as 'apparently recovering fast'. Morton was better and better, and his new surroundings appeared to do him good. But in November of the same year he was not so pliable: he suddenly escaped from Callan Park, then housed at Garryowen, but was quickly picked up by the police. Morton was homesick and lonely, unhappy at his detainment, particularly where it limited his writing career. A month later, he wrote to his brothers in London, suggesting that they were not replying in order to deliberately neglect him.

Morton had reached a plateau in terms of his treatment. At the end of his first year at Callan Park he was confined to his yard – of Ward Two – due to numerous attempts to escape and because he was 'unfit to be at large'. Manning wrote to Fosbery at this time to inform him of Morton's irritability: 'Owing to his escape from the hospital and his expressed intention of again attempting this it has been necessary to keep him under strict surveillance'.[54] As Callan Park was unequipped to deal with such patients, Manning suggested that Morton be moved to Gladesville 'for a change'. While this secondary idea never came to pass, Manning continued to watch Morton's progress, and in April 1882 was still dissatisfied. 'He is extremely discontented,' Manning wrote to Fosbery, and 'has a most exaggerated idea of his own importance and capabilities and is liable to sudden attacks of excitement. I am not without hope that he may in time become much better in mind but at present he would not be safe except in an hospital for the insane'.[55] At this time Morton was refusing to work and fancied 'he [was] utterly lost in both body and soul'. He continued to escape and at one point tried to strangle himself with his neckerchief. At night he was confined by muffs due to a spate of rushes he made on the night attendant in a bid for freedom.

In mid-1882 he began to experience vivid delusions, initially in response to the assassination attempt on Queen Victoria by Roderick MacLean, another writer with his eyes on the position of Poet Laureate. He dreamed that he saw his brother firing at the Queen in MacLean's place. He began to have hallucinations of hearing, which told him to 'blaspheme and curse God Almighty' which he countered with the muttering of prayers under his breath. He also heard voices telling him that if he drank anything he would drown the Virgin Mary who was inside him, or that if he ate anything he would kill someone else; others told him he should stand in the yard, hatless, and pray continually. In December, possessed with the idea that he was his family's guardian, he escaped:

> *George Morton made his escape this afternoon from the cricket paddock between 5pm and 6pm o'clock. He had been out working lately and had given his word that he would not try to escape and was taken to the paddock with the rest of the men by the outdoor attendant Latham. I could not blame Latham very much as the paddock is large and being short-handed there were only two attendants one of whom was playing cricket with the patients. Morton was retaken by the police and handed over to an attendant* [three days later] *who brought him back to hospital.*

Four months later Morton described, in a confiscated letter to his family, the details of this escape, and his frustration at being denied his liberty:

> *... When I escaped from the cricket paddock; I got twenty or so miles off, slept in an Inn for 2/6, had a good breakfast, consisting of cheese, and ten pints of Native Ale, or beer; which, completely set me right; in regard to any weakness, being left in my constitution!!!? It was wrong of me, to drink so much – But you think of my miserable condition; I was taken, fast, asleep; in the Inn – or Tap House; and brought back. I was hand-cuffed, like a felon; stuck up in an open cart; knocked down – set up; and brought back my head now cut open; by an Emissary of the Law in eight (8) places; and I handcuffed; and down – He was a policeman; and I was nowhere. There were besides six men, one mounted with him, so I saw carted*

back; like a dog. Exactly – bound and bleeding in six (6) places from the skull; the blows being struck savagely, with all his force upon my head; – Time: is it not? – That these hellish affairs should be made known to the universe by you? I have been treated and am still, like a Butchered calf; for all the world ...They do not care; being away from the Government and act still, like a set of brutal; savage; infamous; by, MEN –

This letter is one of five which were written by Morton and not sent by the hospital due to the content and his state of mind. Many of them are disturbing in their ideas, and also full of untruths. In January 1883 Morton devoted the first few paragraphs of his letter to his brother with lies about his treatment:

> *How is it you have not written to me for so long?? Are you afraid?? Of what?*
>
> *My health is good – How are you? Are you well??? I thank God I was the happy means of getting you into your Government employ. What we are put into when Children that we should remain. For God is with us AMEN. Have you thought about me in my misery??? What do you think about the Queen's Official Mediciners accusing me of Insanity?????? My Dear Brother I was not insane. I swear it before God I was not Insane when sent here by a Detective:* [illegible]
>
> *My health was Good outside Syphallus. There is little of me left: How can it be otherwise after being two years in hell? For it is hell – No raquet court, no billiard room, no play ground, no Entertainment, no reading Room, no recreation Room, No anything: – To day, I thanks be to God insulted the Head Dr Manning most grossly thank God. He is a Cur: Understan??? := ???:=. A Cur.*
>
> *Dear Rod I can not get out of my misery? Can you help me??? What have you done for me to get me out of here??? ??? ??? –*

Anything???? Why do the Heathen so ferociously rage toegther and why have they murdered the Lords Anointed??? ??? ??? Are you an O'Connor??? And why are you not?????? I cannot understand. It is mysterious. What have they done for you. Have they unmanned you??? ??? ???? Why did you not go to the Queen and demand my liberty??? Oh Ichabod???

These letters were 'unfit for transmission'[56] due to their lies about treatment at Callan Park and fears that the content would distress his recipients. Morton's declarations that he lacked entertainment – naming specific past-times he could not engage in – is interestingly contrary. What Morton named was exactly what he *did* have, and what he would have been encouraged to use and participate in. Such letters were collected by Blaxland and saved for reading and then destruction by Manning, in accordance with the Lunacy Laws.[57] Vast numbers of letters which ought to have been destroyed were kept by the Lunacy Department, but the majority of these were culled in the twentieth century, due to their numbers. It is likely that Morton's were kept due to the nature of his criminal past. It is clear from the content of Morton's letters that he was in constant contact with his family and that the majority of his letters were not kept from being sent. These letters which were kept are fascinating documents in themselves. The first few are decorated with motifs – books, begging hands, little stars and animals – and Morton's flowing handwriting. Interestingly, he signs himself as Arthur O'Connor, and it is hard to imagine that the staff in contact with him – particularly Latham, who figures largely in his complaints about Callan Park – did not know who he really was.

In January 1883 Morton stole his first knife from Ward Two. In 1868 Manning outlined the proper procedure for such implements in the wards:

Table-cloths should be laid, and crockery (plates, mugs, cups, &c.) provided. Tin utensils should be as little used as possible. Ordinary knives, not too sharp, and three-pronged forks, of some common metal, should be allowed, for the majority of the patients, whilst food for the remainder should be cut into small pieces by the attendants, and spoons or forks given to the patients to eat with. Immediately after each meal, all the knives should be collected, counted, and locked up.[58]

All cutlery, in both the communal dining halls at Kirkbride and the individual dining rooms in the wards, was always counted out and back in, to ensure no patient had the opportunity to remove a weapon for later use. Morton secreted his knife out of the Ward Two dining room in the waist of his trousers, which says as much about his cunning as it does the counting skills of the staff of Ward Two. As a result, Morton was made to have his meals separate to the rest of his ward, Blaxland writing that he had 'no good intent'. Blaxland was right to be suspicious, as Morton later explained that the knife had been secreted for the purpose of stabbing the medical superintendent himself, who he erroneously referred to as 'Doctor Blackstone' in his letters. He told Blaxland that he was in Hell 'because I [do] not have your heart's blood'.

The next month another knife went missing, this time found by another patient, the fairly innocuous Merritt, behind the earth box outside in the yard. Morton was still in a bad state at this time, writing again to his mother to complain about his imaginary ill-treatment:

I write to inform you I am not yet discharged – How are you? ... I am very well – In my last letter I informed you about Brooker (Miss) and her conduct toward me, a perfect stranger; this week I write about other things ... I am very well. My appetite is first class. This is a good sign. I sleep very well. – I am in a cell ... This portends very bad. I was put in it by Dr Blackstone [Dr Blaxland]. *I was troubled by religion – and voices. It was all fancy. Caused by the man William Brennan, a Patient, talking religion to me especially about fasting & praying which I did not believe in. He said, I would be 'd'-'d' if I ate. This annoyed me; and brought me down very low-He had great influence over me, through being of a religious turn of mind and I tried to fast; but could, or would not, and my conscience brought me down very low; and I ate – What do you think??? ??? ??? ??? He is a scoundrel; and a reprobate – no more! I am still in a cell; at night. It is horrible? Yes. I have no where to lay my head. And I see & hear not the slightest word as to be shifted. What is to be done??? –*

I am worse than a convict. For he does know his fate:– But I do not. No. The shadow of death is on me; and I am treated as a felon. They cannot deny it. What do they mean by placing me in a cell? To drive me mad with terror? – Every artifice which villainy and fraud could think of, has been tried upon me, by the Government, to drive me raving mad, for ever, but– they don't succeed. No: There are ten thousand pounds, worse patients, here, than me; and they are permitted to sleep in large rooms, with beds, although perfect Demoniacs, and not safe one from another. While I a perfect convalescent from syphallus have to lay in a stone cell by myself and no one within call; If I was to knock till death was on me; It is fearful all through a cur named Brennan, coming here under the pretence of Lunacy. There is not the faintest shadow of release; not the faintest slightest syllable of the Dr being more of a human being, or at least a Gentleman? towards me –

Three months later, however, Morton seemed much better, writing much more coherent and sustained letters. He wrote to his mother in August 1883, worried that patients had seen through his alias, but rather myopically signing this letter, '[your] affectionate son, Arthur O'Connor, Geo Morton, [son of] Madame Catherine O'Connor'. But soon after he was recorded as saying to staff that he could sense a relapse on the horizon, and was quite miserable-looking. In response, he stole a third knife, this time hiding it at the head of his bed. He denied all knowledge of the thing, and 'was very abusive when asked about it'.

The O'Connor family was not overly satisfied with Morton's treatment. Unlike his time at Hanwell, his sanity seemed to rise and fall at Callan

Park and as a result he did not look even close to discharge. The O'Connors acknowledged Morton's clear need for care, but wanted him out of Callan Park. In the grand tradition of the O'Connor family presumption, one of Morton's brothers wrote to the Earl of Derby in 1885 to request permission to send Roderick O'Connor, brother of Morton, to Sydney to care for him. The O'Connors were aware of Morton's insanity but believed it 'to be aggravated by his isolation from any relative or friend and in view of his being a source of trouble to the authorities and to the Government' they believed the situation would be easily remedied by the presence of one of Morton's brothers in Sydney. Roderick would 'watch and protect him [Morton], and be the means of saving the authorities any further trouble'. Of course, such a request was accompanied by a monetary one – the government would need to fund this scheme.[59]

The answer was a negative one. No favours were to be done for Morton – particularly any which might end in his return to England at this stage in his treatment. Of course, Morton continued to attempt escape, eager for a taste of freedom he would never be officially allowed. In August 1885, he vanished while working in the cricket paddock, only to be quickly brought back the next day.

In 1886, in a letter to Manning, Morton seemed to have come to a realisation concerning his ongoing need for care. His tone is one of acceptance, though he was bitter at being removed from the normal rites of passage a young man should experience.

> *Dear Sir,*
> *After being here going on for 6 years my discharge is now it seems put off for heavens only knows how long. I was to have been away by this time according to Dr Blaxland two months ago he said so. I have had the misfortune to be treated with great friendliness and warmth here by a rather engaging young woman a nurse before the season of dancing from whom I was unable to obtain a single dance during the season being simply spurned like a 'damned cur'. The change in the young person was so utter, and incomprehensible that*

at the end of the season I laid up for a couple of days being I suppose a bit worn by the struggle to obtain a little honour and happiness in my miserable position and quite dumbfounded that such a simple pleasure as a dance should have been denied me, like every great and little happiness or benefit which I have sought in my life. Dr Blaxland does not give me the slightest hope of getting out now. I was told that I was 'not a good partner' by and which words I put my own construction upon. The extraordinary demeanour of the creature towards me in the ballroom for 6 months as contrasted with her human words and human behaviour up to the moment of the ball was simply shocking. My opinion is that Miss Paine the nurse was almost speechlessly drunk every dancing night and got so for the deliberate purpose of exasperating me with imbecility and mimic imitation of aristocratic repose, hauteur and patrician [illegible] *for and indifference to inferiority. I suppose the wretched creature was seduced the night before the dances and changed to a heartless fury by it – Dr Blaxland says I can't look at a woman without going wrong. It seems to me that my chances of leaving here are rather dim. I never lost my head. I want to know from you how long this is likely to put me back and when I can confidently look forward to obtaining the blessing of liberty. Can I have the satisfaction of being present at an examination of Miss Paine for drunkeness in the Ballroom. – If I am mistaken in all this, for Christ's sake give me discharge like a man – and let me go.*

In November 1887, Morton made his final mistake. Allowed Sunday parole, an indication of his closeness to discharge due to his ability to care for himself, he did not return to the hospital that evening. The police had to return him the next day. Morton's fate, a lifetime of care, was effectively sealed. He had been in care for six years and showed no sustained indication of any increase in his mental health. He was a chronic patient then, to be managed and contained on a daily basis.

In the medical census of 1890 he was described as being in a 'state of chronic mania'. He was always 'thinking himself ill-used in some way – generally that some woman has trifled with his feelings, he is childish and has great ideas of his looks, intelligence and strength'. In the next few years Morton amused himself by working in the gardens and the attendants' dining room, a plumb job one must assume, and one indicative of his good behaviour. In the early twentieth century he was allowed 'more liberty than most patients', even being allowed to go to Town with attendant H. Carter. Morton had been institutionalised, unable to be of the world outside Callan Park. As the years went on, he became suspicious and nervous around doctors and was moved between Wards Two and One. He was moved eventually to Rydalmere as a chronic patient, then to Morisset and back to Rydalmere. He died in 1925 and was buried at Rookwood under his alias George Morton.

George Morton was not really a criminal – he was an inconvenient person which the British government could not handle because they could not help him. Dr Manning did though, and Morton lived a secure and comfortable life in safety in Blaxland's hospital. Samuel Payne, one of Morton's fellow patients, was not a felon either – but he was under the impression that he was.

8

SAMUEL PAYNE[1]

Guarded by two wardsmen[2] Joseph Thomas Sullivan declared himself, before a packed Melbournian courtroom in mid 1876, to be a mere 'publican now out of business'.[3] A more accurate description might have made reference to the fact that he was a turncoat gang murderer and lately an informant for the New Zealand police.

A few years previously, Sullivan had been a member of the Burgess gang which operated throughout New Zealand.[4] Its leader was Richard Hill. Hill had originally been transported to Australia for theft. While doing his time in the country, Hill had stolen the surname of an Australian man he had attempted to rob and thus re-Christened himself Richard Burgess. Burgess was joined in New Zealand by Thomas Noon who was known to him from time in prison, and who now decided upon the new name of Thomas Kelly. William – really Phillip – Levy was the gang's fence. Finally, there was Sullivan. Originally transported from England to Australia for robbery in 1840, he was now a publican recently having lived in Victoria. Burgess, Kelly, Levy and Sullivan committed various crimes in New Zealand, centred mainly around their forte of robbery, but their exploits came to a head in June 1866.

In 1866, Manning had not yet arrived in Sydney to be greeted by Henry Parkes; Legard was just returning from his second trip to England and about to embark upon his teaching position at Mademoiselle Naegueli's Boarding and Day School; Parcelli was a teenager of fifteen living in Italy and perhaps dreaming of a life in Australia.

On 10 June 1866 the Burgess gang arrived in the gold mining centre of Canvas Town on the Northern most tip of the South Island of New Zealand. They convinced a local shopkeeper, George Jervis, to allow them lodgings. While the others settled into their new accommodation, Levy was instantly dispatched to find a target to rob, ideally someone who had found fortune in the rich earth. Somewhat unwisely, Levy settled upon a publican named Felix Mathieu whom he had met before. Mathieu was part of a group of men readying themselves for a journey to the West Coast. Mathieu, James Dudley, John Kempthorne and James de Pontius were ripe targets: they carried with them a large amount of money and gold excavated from the soil of Canvas Town.

The Burgess gang's plan was simple: ambush Mathieu and his friends and relieve them of their wealth. But such a plan could not be carried out within the town itself; the Burgess gang would risk arrest in such a small town and with so many potential witnesses. They decided to wait until the four marks had left for the West Coast and were travelling. They would be alone, and there would be no one to either interrupt or observe the crime on the track. Burgess and his accomplices left the town earlier than Mathieu and his friends on the morning in question, resolving to travel ahead of them and then lie in wait for them to come along the road. Then they would attack.

The first aspect of the plan which went wrong was the meeting of a potential witness on the road. The gang had counted on the track being relatively quiet, and thus free of witnesses to place them in the location of a robbery once the alarm was raised and they were fleeing. Early on their journey along the track soon to be trod by their victims, they passed a man named James Battle. Concerned that Battle might come to assist the police in tracking them down after the robbery had been committed, the Burgess gang decided that he was too dangerous a witness. Rather than abandon their plan, they killed him and robbed him of £3. After Burgess and Sullivan had strangled him, they buried him on the side of the track. The grisly task having been completed, the four secreted themselves near the summit of the Maungatapu Track and waited for Mathieu and his friends to ride by, gold in their saddle bags.

They did not have long to wait, and soon Mathieu and his friends rode into the trap that had been set for them. Mathieu was first, being stabbed and shot; Dudley was strangled; Kempthorne, de Pontius and their packhorse, which carried £320 worth of gold and cash, were all shot. The deed done, Sullivan and his thugs fled with riches in their pockets.

But just after the murderers had divided up the spoils and dispersed from the scene of four hasty burials, a friend of Mathieu's rode by. Henry Moller, who had been expecting to meet his friends at some point on the track, and aware of the cargo they had with them, was worried by their absence. He must have ridden right past their graves. When he arrived in Nelson and found they were missing, he alerted the police. The police focused their investigation on Canvas Town where they had been last seen alive, and their suspicions quickly settled on shopkeeper Jervis' odd visitors. By 19 June, all four members of the Burgess gang had been rounded up and arrested.

Finding some evidence of a crime, the police were still uncertain as to exactly what had occurred and offered approximately £200 and a free pardon to anyone who turned Queen's evidence. Stoic and with some experience of police interrogation, Burgess, Kelly and Levy held their tongues but Sullivan jumped at the opportunity to condemn his colleagues and save his own skin. Portraying himself as an unhappy accomplice, Sullivan declared himself merely a lookout for the thugs and identified Burgess as the terrifying and persuasive ringleader of the gang. The police had a result: the fear gripping the West Coast of New Zealand would finally dissipate. The bodies were located and given proper burials. Burgess, Kelly and Levy were tried for the murder of the Mathieu party. It took the jury less than an hour to find them guilty of murder. Sullivan's turncoat antics provided for him an amnesty which protected him from even being charged.

The gang were hanged. Burgess was said to have kissed his noose as he stood on the platform from which he was to be executed. He told the waiting crowd that 'he had no more fear of death than he had of going to a wedding'. Kelly, who had cried when his sentence had been handed down, had to be carried to his noose; Levy continued to protest his innocence even until the last.

The murder of James Battle, however, was a separate issue, and Sullivan found that the amnesty which protected him from punishment for the Mathieu party's murders did not apply here. He was put on trial for the murder and the jury, ever consistent, needed very little time to find him guilty. He was sentenced to death. But here the police intervened: what future criminal would turn Queen's evidence on the promise of protection, if they saw Sullivan now abandoned? The public were outraged: Sullivan was a dangerous murderer and should not avoid punishment. His death sentence was commuted to life imprisonment[5] and Sullivan became a feared figure in the public consciousness.

In early 1868 Sullivan found himself a prisoner in Dunedin Gaol, readying himself for a lifetime of incarceration but protected from the angry and fearful public. But the police were still caught with a difficult prisoner: life in prison was not so very different to death to future turncoats and so in 1874 he was pardoned – and like Morton – on the condition that he never return to New Zealand. Sullivan chose initially to forsake his family and instead return to England, his mother country, and where he had been first arrested and punished with transportation. But by the end of the year he was in Australia, trying to get back to his wife and two children who were caretakers for his freehold property in Victoria. If Victoria was sensitive about lunatics arriving by boat, it was seriously concerned about criminals arriving at its ports and setting up their lives. Sullivan was arrested upon arrival under the Influx of Criminals Prevention Act and imprisoned in Melbourne Gaol.

Sullivan's presence in Australia was alarming: he was not just a killer but a dishonourable one. He could kill with his bare hands – had a trail of five dead men behind him, plus those of his fellow gang members – and had during his life been known as a prize fighter. He was an intimidating and unnerving figure in the public consciousness. Even more disturbing was the Victorian government's inability to keep him in prison: Sullivan's lawyer argued in court that because his client had been domiciled in Victoria *before* the passing of the Act, he was consequently exempt.[6] As a result, Sullivan was released into society, striking fear into not just the Victorian, but Australian, population.

A quiet man-hunt began: Sullivan was not guilty of any new crime, but the newspapers of the day portrayed the public's obsession with him. Numerous sightings were constantly made of Sullivan, and he appears to have been driven out of various small townships all over Australia. The unspoken aim was to make him as unwelcome as possible and focus so much attention on him as to make it impossible for him to kill again. A week after his release, he was sighted in Ballarat.[7] Another week later an article appeared in the *Wagga Wagga Advertiser* claiming Sullivan's crimes were worse than originally thought, and that Australian lives had been taken by him along with those of New Zealanders':

> *Now that the murderer Sullivan occupies a prominent place in the public mind, it is worth while retrieving a story that has previously been narrated, and which has all the elements of probability within it. Dr King, JP., informs us (says a Ballarat paper), that about fifteen years ago, his brother, residing at Korong, in the vicinity of Sullivan's shanty, was firmly impressed with the belief that Sullivan was then engaged in the fiendish work of murder... Sullivan owned a grog shop at Korong, into which several men, with money, were induced to enter, who have never since been heard of. The supposition then was that the men received poison in their grog. The hypothesis, or, as the gentleman named regard it, certainty, as to the disposal of the bodies is, that they were buried in the garden. Sullivan, it is said, was in the habit of trenching his land to the extraordinary depth of four feet, and this business he only carried on at night. He also strewed the trenches with bones of animals, and the view held by Dr King, his brother, and others was, that this precaution was taken against the discovery of human bones.*[8]

Sullivan was still in Australia a year on and continued to inspire the same kind of fear he had when he had first set foot upon Victorian soil:

On last Monday evening a stranger arrived at Cootamundra and stayed for a while at Mr Angrove's Hotel, where he was supplied with tea. After he had partaken of this he adjourned to the bar, where the effects of the beer, of which he had often and largely imbibed, soon began to make him talkative. In answer to several, he stated that he was Gately, the Melbourne hangman. He was then asked if he had ever been in NZ. He replied, 'Yes: he knew more of NZ than of NSW.' On further enquiry he was recognised as Sullivan, the New Zealand murderer. As I am given to understand he is making towards Yass, I forward a description of his appearance at the time I saw him on Monday night: – He is a strong, powerfully built man, about six foot in height. I should say his age is over 50; he is very dark-complexioned, with black hair; Newgate kind of shave, with a little tuft of black air on chin, and altogether possesses a most forbidding countenance. He was dressed in an old coat ... a dirty coloured shirt, mole trousers, dirty red comforter, and an old black hat, with a towel round it for a turban. As soon as he found his identity was discovered he made tracks and has not been seen here since. On Tuesday morning there was a great many people on the alert to catch a glimpse of him, but he had fled during the night. I am given to understand that the police kept a strict watch over him until he left the town. There is not the faintest doubt that he is Sullivan, for he was recognised by a man who had seen him in New Zealand. The visitor stated that he was come from New Zealand and was making his way to Sydney with a view to take ship for England – Correspondent Yass Courier.[9]

An exact description was something which was of paramount importance in the public mind – how else would one be able to protect oneself? One writer for the *Evening News*[10] begged to differ with the acknowledged description of Sullivan:

> *A correspondent 'who has had the pleasure of seeing Sullivan on several occasions,' writes to the* Yass Courier, *to say that our correspondent at Cootamundra 'made a mistake with regard to the description of the gentleman called Sullivan, the New Zealand murderer.' He adds – 'I have been in New Zealand from 1862 to 1870, and have had the pleasure of seeing him on several occasions. He is not six feet high, nor has he black hair. He has grey hair, round smooth-shaved face, about five feet nine inches in height. He was in my house about five weeks ago, and I asked him in the presence of several parties how New Zealand looked, when he left here at once, and went towards Jerilderie.'*

In this atmosphere of fear and suspicion, perpetuated primarily by the newspapers of the colony, a man named Samuel Payne became very unwell.

Payne was an English labourer who had lived in Forbes for some years when in mid-1877 he began to hear voices in his head telling him he was Sullivan 'the New Zealand murderer'. This internal insistence deeply disturbed Payne and was probably initiated by his local newspaper, the journalists for which had made a connection between the circulating images of Sullivan and the appearance of Payne. The police, who were on the lookout for men fitting Sullivan's description, agreed with the journalists. Samuel Payne found that his house was being watched by the suspicious local police and that local residents had been 'warned' about him.

This alienation from the rest of his community deeply injured Payne and he began to exhibit signs of melancholia. Likely unwell for some time, this change in circumstances exacerbated his condition and he fell into a deep depression. Worse, he began to believe the newspaper reports and the rumours circulating about him: he began to believe that he *was* Sullivan. Being watched as he was, Payne's symptoms were noted and in October 1877 he was arrested for the crime of 'unsound mind' and taken to Bathurst Gaol. He had with him £2 5s, a pair of scissors, two knives, a pocket book, a purse and some matches. In a clear case of insanity, Payne was not taken first to Reception House; instead, he was transferred directly to Gladesville.

At Gladesville Payne was summarised as a forty-nine-year-old labourer. He was diagnosed as suffering from a delusional melancholia caused by a 'lonely life'. He was suicidal – particularly as he believed himself culpable for the murders of the Mathieu party in New Zealand along with James Battle – also sullen, sleepless, suffering from delusions of hearing and in poor physical health. In a moment rather lacking in sympathy, there was an unhelpful note made at the start of his pages in the *Medical Case Book* adding, 'He is a tall ugly dark-complexioned man whose appearance may easily be mistaken for a murderer'. Such matter-of-fact cruelties were not unusual in Callan Park's files at this time.

Two years at Gladesville had little effect on Payne: he was usually well-conducted and 'useful but very delusionally insane'. At other times he was characterised as 'very idle and makes no change'. Though generally quiet, he was sometimes 'sulky, sullen and angry looking', and constantly demanding his discharge. He called Gladesville a prison – Payne was not the only one to do so, as he struggled to come to terms with his need for supervision while undergoing treatment – and continued to suffer 'hallucinations of hearing'.

In December 1879 he was transferred out of Gladesville to Callan Park in the same group which Chan Long, Joshua Fitzpatrick and James Daniel Webster were a part of. His first act was to 'join in' on the attack initiated by Parcelli, Clancy and Legard on the Ward Two attendants, for which he was secluded with his fellow assailants. Aside from this initial act, Payne quickly found peace at Callan Park. After a couple of months in the weatherboard buildings beside Garryowen it was remarked that while he 'retains his fancies [he] does not often give expression to them', a sure indication that improvement was being made. The electric lights scared him however, and he was frightened that their real use was not to illuminate the rooms but to 'see into his past life'. His second full year at Callan Park, 1881, was characterised by an increase in violence directed at other patients, and a high level of idleness. In 1882 he began to assist more in the wards, applying himself to the job of painting. But his delusions quickly retuned as he worked and he was forced to stop.

In 1885, Payne appeared to turn a corner again. He started working in the engine room – but it was quickly realised that he would not be consistent in this, and when he *did* work it was only to make a show of his strength. The medical staff at Callan Park were not fooled and in a census carried out in 1890, where every patient was examined, Payne was bluntly described as one who 'suffers from Chronic Mania – has delusions of persecution by electricity ... mutters incoherently ... good humoured but lazy ... mak[es] a pretence of assisting in the engine house'. This census was initiated to cleanse Callan Park of its chronic patients, and transfer these to asylums then ear-marked for long-stay patients. Payne was one of these men: chronic and unlikely to be ever discharged. He was removed to Kenmore in Goulburn where he continued to be cared for along with the likes of Parcelli. Kenmore's files having been lost, and the Inspector General of the Insane's *Registers* not always kept updated, it is unclear why – and when – Payne was discharged from Kenmore and came to be buried elsewhere than at Kenmore's private cemetery.

Whatever the cause, Samuel Payne was likely buried at Rookwood in November 1921 in an unmarked pauper's grave on the very edge of the cemetery. A visitor today might easily mistake the wide overgrown field for an empty one; but the tall grass and thousands of wild flowers have a charm about them and stand as a moving monument to this friendless labourer from Forbes who thought he was Joseph Sullivan.

9

ESCAPEES[1]

Escapes – sometimes pre-meditated but often opportunistic – were an issue to be dealt with in all asylums. After all, institutions with predictable routines are open to this kind of abuse even today. When Garryowen House only was home to Callan Park Hospital for the Insane, a huge number of escapes occurred with patients scaling the short paling fences at opportune times such as the changeover of staff or just prior to meal times, much to the frustration of Blaxland. The fear of being harassed or attacked by an escapee loomed large in the public consciousness at this time – and was one of the arguments residents in the vicinity of Callan Park used to try to block the use of Garryowen as a hospital for the insane. Indeed, the *Annual Reports* from Manning reflected this public interest, and numbered the escapes from each institution each year, with statistics concerning the number of recaptures versus the number who found permanent liberation.

But escapes were not about attacking members of the public – they were about personal freedom, or the ecstasy of actually *running*. For the most part they represented an opportunity for a taste of freedom or, more likely a taste of beer, and only lasted for a few hours. Only occasionally did an escape indicate the unhappiness of a patient; more often they cast light onto the ineptness of the staff member employed to keep an eye on patients who seemed to regard escape as an interesting way to break the monotony of life in care. Fear of staff and treatment did not seem to be an initiating factor in the escapes at early Callan Park: patients seemed rather desirous of the adrenaline of the pursuit. Callan Park's issue was not so much concerned with the escapees themselves

– very, very few were never returned to the hospital – but rather in the *cost* of the manpower required to return the escapee.

Of course, preventative measures were taken at all of Manning's hospitals to try to limit the numbers of men – and women – vanishing during the day and night. Patients who formed working parties around the grounds of the asylum were counted out and then back into their ward by the attendants, at the end of the work. Even single patients being escorted back to their wards were required to be 'signed in' by the staff member with them, to ensure that the ward attendants were aware the patient had returned. The vigilance of all staff – even the artisans, servants and gardeners – was also needed, and all staff were required to report suspicious behaviour to the attendants in charge of the wards.

Probably the best measure by which nocturnal escapes were controlled was by the locking up of patients' clothes at night. Only convalescent patients with clean records were allowed a chest within which they might keep their clothes.[2] Occasionally, however, patients managed to keep their trousers – the most valuable article of their wardrobe – through some underhand means. This enabled escape since it meant one would not have the social handicap, particularly after the sun had risen, of lacking pants. E. Fitzpatrick used such a find to good use on two occasions before Blaxland had him transferred to Gladesville. A patient in 1885, Webb, escaped from the Kirkbride Complex, after having collected various tools for the job:

> *... last night Webb attempted to escape. He managed to secrete a large nail which he used as a screwdriver and removed the wooden stops placed to prevent the upper sash of the window from being opened more than a certain distance. He then pulled down the sash, got onto the balconette to which he attached his sheet and lowered himself onto the verandah roof and passed round till he came to the dividing wall along which he proceed till he reached the plantation facing nos i and ii wards; two attendants who had just returned home heard him walking along the roof and guessing the direction he could take, were waiting for him in the plantation. He*

had a pair of trousers on when retaken which belonged to another patient who had secreted them in the night commode. The attempt was made just after the 10 o'clock rounds ...

Single rooms also helped combat these night-time adventures, as they minimised the patients' abilities to work in teams to find escape, and had lockable shutters over the windows.

In the event that a patient did actually manage to get away from the hospital, many frequently returned of their own free will. Hunger, loneliness, disorientation and the sudden realisation that the world outside the bounds of the hospital was a busy and uncaring place, forced many to reverse their ideas of freedom and re-arrive in their ward. This is one of the strongest aspects which implied that patients were well treated under Blaxland: even the insane would be reluctant to return to a place of barbarism and torture. Sometimes patients were brought back by attendants, sometimes they were returned by the police, who were always notified in the event of an escape, and sometimes by strangers who recognised the patient by their manner and clothes. Manning disliked the idea of a uniform for patients, saying that such uniformity 'can be desirable only as a check upon escape from the asylum, and its disadvantages much outweigh the trifling advantage which is gained'.[3] Instead, he opted for colourful, patterned clothes as the general public might wear, but which were marked with the words 'Callan Park'.

Aside from all this, however, was the law. If a patient escaped from their hospital and could not be retrieved within twenty-eight days, then they were automatically discharged and struck off the books. Manning's staff could not be expected to search for these men and women in perpetuity. If a patient managed to remove him or herself from the asylum and make his or her own way in the world – finding accommodation and work, thus being able to function normally outside the walls of the asylum – then that patient was not hunted or harassed. To the contrary: it meant that Manning and Blaxland, and indeed all of the staff, had done their job and cured the patient. Such an event was one of success and a cause for celebration. In 1881 John Denison, a convalescent patient on the verge of official discharge by Blaxland, did just that, and after the twenty-eight days had elapsed, contacted Callan Park to declare that he was well and employed.[4] Justice Sipple,[5] a tall German melancholic who had suffered fits from the age of eleven and delusions of persecution which resulted in his committal at Gladesville in 1876, did the same as Denison in 1888 and was never heard of again.

One of the finest escapees at early Callan Park was Alexander Clubb.[6] Born in 1848 in Scotland to John Clubb and Ann Newlands, Alexander – who preferred 'Alex' to 'Alexander' – was one of several children in the Clubb household. In 1851 they were recorded as living in Fochabers, Moray: John, thirty-two, a plasterer; Ann, thirty; Ann, ten, a scholar; Eliza, seven, a scholar; George, four; Alexander, two, with John, their final child, born some years later. In 1852 the extensive Clubb family arrived on the *Bermondsey* in New South Wales and settled in the Balmain area, making them neighbours of the area which was to become Callan Park.

The *Balmain Directory* for 1879 – the same year Alex was committed – recorded him as working as a plasterer, like his father, and living in Nelson Street in Balmain. George, his older brother, was described as living nearby in Beattie Street, a plastering contractor. John, the youngest brother, was living in Ewell Street, with their father, John Snr, listed as a plasterer living at Merton Cottage in Darling Road. The Clubbs appear in this list to have been a picture of family felicity: successful immigrants working their trade.

But what the *Balmain Directory* did not show was the crumbling mental state of Alex Clubb, youngest but one. An unusual candidate for institutional care in New South Wales at this time due to his strong family support, in May 1879 Clubb arrived at the Central Police Office, probably under arrest rather than merely having been escorted there by a concerned family member. His arrival at the Police Office tends to indicate that there was some kind of incident connected to his being taken to Reception House, since concerned family members did not need to go through the police: the mentally unwell could just as easily be taken directly to Reception House, thus bypassing the police – and associated fuss – entirely. Being described as twenty-nine years old, rather than the correct thirty-one years which could easily have been recorded by a member of his extensive family, also indicated he was brought in by strangers who estimated his personal details. After his transfer to Darlinghurst Clubb was at Reception House for the comparatively long time of almost a week during which time he oscillated between quietness, and restlessness and fretfulness. His father at some point in this time visited him, and signed his blue warrant papers for 'conveyance to a madhouse'.

The obvious place for Clubb was at Callan Park, so as to be near his family, but at this time – May 1879 – Callan Park was readying itself for the first influx of new patients to be added to the first forty-four and was not in a position to take any new patients who required a large degree of supervision. So Clubb was registered at Gladesville, the next closest asylum to his Balmain-based family.

Gladesville's stance appears to have been to merely contain Clubb; he was ear-marked for transfer to Callan Park as soon as this could be arranged, and a result he was not closely monitored in his first five months of care. The staff entered his father's details as his next of kin in their books, and there was a note recording the fact that John Clubb had been notified of his son's removal to Callan Park in October 1879. While at Gladesville Clubb was restless, as he had been at Reception House. He was 'given to absurd gesticulations and suffered from considerable impediment of speech'. He was plagued by religious delusions, but his incoherent speech did not allow for close study or understanding of these. At times he was erratic and described, unusually for Gladesville where staff usually tried to put a positive spin on all behaviour, as 'unmanageable'. A note at the end of this description added that even though his bodily health had improved, his mental health had not altered at all.

Clubb arrived at Garryowen House as a member of the third group of twelve patients who increased the ranks of the insane in New South Wales' newest asylum. He was a member of the most disturbed group to arrive at the new hospital – part of a transfer which included Fillipo Parcelli, William Andrews, William Clancy and Henry Jollis. In his notes he was described as having in the last two years been subject to a developing mania. Questions relating to his suicidal tendencies and danger to others were answered in the affirmative. Clubb had never been admitted to any hospital before, and had no insane relations. He was installed in Ward Two as a paying patient. His father and later his brother George, when his father had passed away, paid 15s and 2d per month for his care.

Staff at Callan Park found Clubb initially to be 'flighty and incoherent' but not 'troublesome'. In a few more months they discovered his delusions centred partly on the Queen, and some 'very exalted notions of his own rank'. Despite these, he worked well in the wards and was described as 'industrious'. Callan Park's *Visitor Record* no longer exists, but it cannot be doubted that Clubb's family were frequent visitors during this time, living so near. Of relevance is also the lack of complaints made by his family concerning his treatment. The fact that the relatives of patients at Callan Park generally had no concerns speaks, again, highly of Blaxland and his staff. It was not lost on Clubb that he was in Balmain, the place in which he had effectively grown up after his departure from Scotland, and after the initial period where he settled into his new surrounds, Clubb began his escaping spree.

In 1882 Clubb was working with attendant Love, the same staff member who had been involved in the spraining of Legard's leg the previous year. Love, not always being the most scrupulously careful of patients, but never actively violent, 'took Clubb with him to empty some slops into the pig's bucket and instead of going to the bucket with him stayed at the kitchen; when he thought Clubb ought to have returned he went to look for him and on finding he had escaped, gave notice, but nothing could be found of him.' Clubb was elusive – most likely a fit and agile ex-plasterer and still quite young, he was a man made to escape. Blaxland was not impressed: the supervision of patients even in small jobs like this was paramount. But like so many of his fellow escapees, Clubb's escape left himself at a loss. He appeared not to have gone to any of his siblings, but instead walked around Balmain for the remainder of the day on his own. The next morning, when the police were also at a loss for the vanishing patient, Clubb inexplicably 'walked into Attendant [George] Bulfin's house for a drink of water' and the attendant 'being at home brought him back to hospital.' Blaxland was relieved but angry, writing in the hospital's *Journal*, 'I consider Love to blame in not going the whole distance with Clubb, however as it was his first offence he was left off with a caution'. Attendants lived on site at Callan Park, often with their families. It is difficult to imagine any ill treatment of Clubb by Bulfin while in his house, quite possibly with his young family present.

The object of Clubb's multiple escapes is unclear. Many patients left their ward with purpose: for an unrestricted drinking session in a pub, to see their families, and in one instance, to attempt to find a lawyer to plead their case of sanity. But Clubb seems to have had no motivation other than to accept the challenge of the quick escape. He was not the only one: in the same year Charles Gibson, a patient who earlier had needed restraint by muffs to stop him putting his fingers down his throat to induce vomiting, escaped from Ward Three:

> *Charles Gibson made his escape today just before dinner hour from no iii ward, he took advantage of the attendant working in the flower bed. He was missed at dinner time and efforts were made to retake him which however were not successful until 7pm when he was returned to hospital by the gardener near whose house he wandered. I can scarcely blame the attendant as the fence is easily scaled and this patient has on many other occasions attempted to get over and was brought back before effecting his purpose.*

Clubb did it again later in 1882, when he vanished from Ward Two at some point between 4pm and 6pm. The fact he was not missed until tea-time speaks of the occasional lack of supervision in Ward Two. Blaxland, again recording the event, wrote that 'no trace could be found of him and his mode of escape remains a mystery as none of the attendants know anything about it nor as far as can be ascertained do any of the patients.' The police were informed and Blaxland waited for news. An entry was made in the *Police Gazette,*[7] describing Clubb as five feet ten inches tall, with a dark complexion, dark hair and beard and moustache, and brown eyes. He was dressed in cord trousers, a light tweed jumper and drab soft felt hat, and boots with buckles. He was missing for twelve days – setting the record for early Callan Park – until senior constable Day of the Sydney police arrested him and handed him over to the Balmain police.[8] Arriving back in Ward Two, he was pleased to explain his mode of escape: he 'slipped through' with other patients who were being taken by attendant Carter to the cricket paddock – that haven for the potential escape artist – and jumped the short fence to freedom. Carter, though sometimes not the most observant of the staff, was defended by Blaxland, who could not believe that Carter would have overlooked Clubb. A question mark was placed over Clubb's version of events.

Clubb was to remain in care until his death. There was no major alteration in his mental state during the rest of his life. He worked well as a wardsman in Ward Two, assisting the staff. Sometimes he was abusive and violent. Alex Clubb died in 1919 of heart disease and was buried at Rookwood near the entry to the cemetery. Unlike so many of Callan Park's patients, Clubb was mourned – by his brother.

But not every patient was struck by a crushing lack of direction or purpose after effecting his escape. For some this was a serious business and they were determined to go to ground once out, and to gain the twenty-eight days of freedom needed to begin their new lives. While this was deemed acceptable for patients such as Sipple and Denison, who were convalescent and likely to be able to care for themselves, other patients were not in such a healthy position and Callan Park was obliged to begin a serious search for them.

In 1883 there were two major escapes from Garryowen House, both from associated dormitories. The first involved a group of three dangerous men: William Williams (alias Crook), William Swain (alias Henry Williams)[9] and Paul Littel who worked together to achieve their escape. Crook was an English labourer in his early thirties, suffering from a delusional mania. His beliefs centred mainly on religion and an unjust persecution by the police – his acting on the latter having brought him to Manning's institution:

> *He is reported to have complained to Bishop Barker that the police at Nundle had unlawfully imprisoned him for two days and that subsequent to this, finding things disagreeable in the neighbourhood he came down to Sydney when he went to the Inspector General of police who gave him in charge as of unsound mind.*

Crook was to spend a lifetime in care, going eventually to Rydalmere as a chronic patient in 1894.

Paul Littel, a twenty-seven-year-old German who had worked as a gardener in Prussia, was also diagnosed as a delusional maniac, cause unknown. He was described as being 'a young man of good manners', which was consistent with his delusions which centred around his having been sent to New South Wales for 'some political office'. His fancies told him that Queen Victoria had made him governor of New South Wales, and his time at Callan Park was marked by repeated instances in which he asked for leave to visit Her Majesty. By 1882, a year into his care, Littel was a keen assistant in the gardens at Callan Park, and probably played a major role in readying those attached to the Kirkbride Complex. He was also convinced that he was the King of England by this stage. He made his first escape in the same year:

> [He] *climbed over the roof this morning at attendants' breakfast time (7.30 am). He ran past the carpenter's shop and the carpenter being within saw, gave chase and captured him before he got outside the boundary fence. Two attendants were in the ward at the time and ought to have seen Littel getting on the roof but as he is always watching for a chance he probably took very little time over it. As blame could not be attached to any particular attendant I* [Blaxland] *spoke to both and warned them to take better care in the future.*

In the second half of 1882,

> *An effort was made by the German Consul to send* [Littel] *to Germany and he was sent to Sydney to see if the Ship's Surgeon would pass him. He was so troublesome in the Sydney streets however, proclaiming himself King of Australia and appealing to passers-by that it was necessary to call the assistance of the police once or twice and he was with difficulty brought back to hospital after which it was decided to try no more. The Ship's Surgeon did*

not see him. [Littel also] *imagines there are secret passages under the hospital, by means of which people enter to murder patients nightly also that human flesh is given them to eat.*

In early 1883, a few months before his infamous escape with Crook and Swain, Littel struck Blaxland in the face with an open hand. As his time in care progressed, so did the seriousness of his delusions: by late 1883 he was proclaiming himself Queen of Italy and upon that basis refused to wear a hat. By 1884 he was described as 'very insane' and that he 'says sometimes he is a queen or a princess and at others a Pope or Czar'; he 'assumes a fresh name every now and then and gets very angry if called by his true name'. Like Crook, Littel was a life patient and was transferred to Kenmore in 1907.

Crook and Littel were mere assistants in their vanishing act of 1883: their ringleader was William Swain. Swain was an English 'dealer'. At the time of his escape he was the eldest of the three at thirty-six years old. At home he had a wife and no children. Suffering from mania like Crook and Littel, he was described as having a 'wild expression of countenance'. Untidy and incoherent, he spoke much to himself and 'walk[ed] about constantly'. Like so many, his delusions focused on a wrong done him: for Swain, it was that someone in 'England [had] killed his mother and that they [had] robbed him of the property and that he [was] forced constantly to 'intercede' in the case'. His care at Callan Park included blistering, and he complained of a pain in his limbs and head, and during some periods could not walk. He frequently lied and was labelled as very troublesome.

These three, accommodated perhaps unwisely in an associated dormitory of several men, combined to escape in June 1883. At about 9pm one evening the night attendant Greer was due to come through the dormitory to check all was still and quiet. Instead of passing through the dorm he was lazy and merely peered through one of the windows. Like many attendants, Greer's mistakes were down to benignity rather than violence. Satisfied all was fine, he moved on without proper inspection. As Blaxland would come to record, 'Had [Greer] done [his job] he would in all probability have prevented the escape'. As the light faded from Greer's lamp, as he moved on, the three were up and preparing for their escape. The other patients, who can scarcely be believed to have slept through these moments in the dorm, were also complicit. Greer long gone, Swain and Williams began by wrenching off the iron bar which guarded the lower part of the window when open. If their fellow patients had not been awake before, they were then. Littel assisted Swain in breaking into the clothes press where their clothes were kept overnight. Quickly dressing himself in the dark, Swain despaired out of the window. Left with both the window wide and the clothes press open, Littel and Crook followed him soon after. Soon it was 10pm and Greer was back and armed with a closer attention to detail than previously. He saw the broken window, the clothes press open; the alarm was raised.

Unhappily for the attendants, several were dispatched into the dark Sydney suburbs to find the three fugitives. Swain, the instigator, was captured at midnight by hospital staff probably since his muscle degeneration meant his walking was much impaired; but Littel and Crook remained at large. The next morning Littel, convinced of his importance in New South Wales and the realm, was arrested at Government House where he had tried to gain entrance. Despite his clothes being marked with the clear indictors of his being an asylum patient he was charged by the police as being of unsound mind and taken to the Water Police Court. He was remanded in Reception House for a week. Blaxland encountered, bizarrely, a large amount of difficulty in persuading the magistrates to convey Littel back to Callan Park. When he finally made the police understand that Littel was *already* a patient at Callan Park, Greer was charged the 84d needed to bring Littel back to Balmain. Three days later Crook was taken by the Marulan police and escorted back to hospital. A mere month later, Swain was off again, this time breaking out of a single room (the result of his prior escape) by breaking one of the wooden vents over the door. When stopped and questioned, he denied all knowledge of how the damage had come to be and laid the blame at the feet of some unknown fellow patient determined to get him into trouble.

Attendant Greer was not the only staff member to be reprimanded after an escape. In 1882 outdoor attendant Sloan left patient John Gordon (a different Gordon to Garryowen's previous owner) alone in the grounds 'while he went to defecate'. Seizing this opportunity, Gordon disappeared and was 'pursued but without success' by the recently-relieved and highly-embarrassed Sloan. The next day when Gordon was returned by the police it was noticed that he was wearing a coat – which he had not been wearing when he had left – along with 18d in the pocket. When asked, Gordon replied that he had had some clothes in a boarding house which he had gone to pick up and sell. Surprisingly, Blaxland took Sloan's side: 'It was difficult to blame Sloan much but he had to pay the cost of bringing the patient from Sydney'.

The following year Sloan was in trouble again: this time he had taken patient John Barragay (alias Ryan, alias Scully) in order to dig a hole for the night soil. The other attendant in charge, Trevor, arrived to find the hole dug but Barragay missing. Instead of alerting staff to this he made chase on his own but failed to recover the patient. Sloan, though implicated, escaped significant punishment again, but Trevor was obliged to pay a portion of the cost of expense of retaking the patient, who was in the end found by Parramatta police. Barragay, like Clubb, was a serial escapee. A middle-aged labourer from Ireland, with chronic mania, Barragay believed 'the priest of Penrith' was his father. He was prone to sudden outbursts and was described as having a weak intellect. A year after the night-soil incident, he vanished again:

> *Yesterday morning* [Barragay] *made his escape from the gardener under the following circumstances. He was left gathering up some manure near the Entrance gate while the gardener took a load to the garden and on his return found that* [Barragay] *had completed his job and decamped. Several attendants were despatched in pursuit and tho they heard of him along the road to Petersham failed to overtake him. A telegram was sent to the Parramatta police who replied about 7.30pm saying the patient had been retaken; an attendant was sent for him as soon as possible and returned about 1am this morning. The gardener was to blame for leaving* [him] *at work by himself but thought he had enough work to keep him employed till his return; as on each former occasion he escaped,* [he] *finished his job first. Gardener to pay 24 pence of recapture.*

In 1884 he was gone again, departing suddenly from the orchard. He was picked up by staff at Burwood.

But if Sloan and Greer were careless, attendants Hughes, Emerson and Jones were downright slack. In 1886, a convalescent patient named William Jones, being of good behaviour, was allowed to sit up until 8pm (rather than 7pm) by attendant Hughes. Blaxland recorded that William Jones 'was left in the day room or else the doors were left unlocked and he slipped back and made his escape by removing the stops (wood) which prevent the windows opening more than a certain height, from one of the windows from thence he easily scaled the wall. Hughes an attendant being responsible was fined for carelessness'. The previous year attendant Emerson and attendant Jones, both new to their jobs at Callan Park, failed to notice the sudden absence of Michael Summers, a teenager with delusional melancholia. They maintained that they 'saw nothing unusual' the whole afternoon in their ward. Emerson and Jones escaped themselves with only a verbal caution.

Not every attendant got away with a mere caution. One evening in 1889 when convalescent patient William Boyd asked attendant Broadbent for the keys to his ward so that he could get himself a drink of water, he probably couldn't believe his luck when they were handed over. Bypassing his drink, Boyd let himself out of his ward and walked all the way to Gladesville Hospital where he gave himself up to the medical superintendent there and handed over the keys. Broadbent, who had dramatically compromised patient safety, was immediately suspended and dismissed the following morning.

Of course, there were some aspects of Callan Park which invited escape and for which Blaxland could hardly hold his staff responsible. Many patients, including George Morton, found the cricket paddock all too alluring as an easy path to freedom since it sat alongside Balmain Road. A patient, J. Caus, felt the same way one day in 1883, rushing through a bathroom door as his ward was being cleaned out, climbing a shower bath pipe and squeezing through a fan light. From there he ran to the cricket paddock, naked, and with intentions of escaping from there – but was tackled to the ground. Guiseppe Vallos continued the tradition in 1885 and was at large for two weeks until he was retaken by the Sydney police. Windows were also one of Callan Park's weaknesses, with most escapes being made through these despite blocks on how far they could be opened. In a rare note about facilities recorded by Blaxland in the asylum's *Journal*, he wrote in 1882: 'It has been necessary to use restraint somewhat frequently during the past week but chiefly at night in the case of one or two patients who persist in breaking the windows of their single rooms with a view of escaping or attempting suicide. The windows are of glass and I think it will be necessary to substitute with grating in several'. In 1883 D. Brown cut his hands on glass while attempting to escape and was fitted with a camisole to prevent any further harm; in 1886 Robert Scott,

> *escaped from a single room soon after 12 midnight. By some means unknown he opened the railway lock of the shutters and having broken the stop of the sash got thro the window, scaled the wall of the yard and made off towards Petersham with his clothing but his shirt. He was stopped by two civilians and handed over to the police who at once returned him to the hospital after an absence of about half an hour ... no blame attaches to any of the attendants.*

In the same year patient Winders '... was allowed to sit up till 8 o'clock at night and having asked to be allowed to go into the WC effected his escape by climbing through the fanlight over the door leading into the yard. There was certainly some carelessness on the part of the attendants in charge but the window is unnecessarily large and will be replaced by wire grating'.

The majority of Callan Park's runaways were swiftly returned, either by the police or hospital staff who seemed to be permanently ready to give chase, or by members of the public. Callan Park's *Journals* and *Case Books* are full of irate gardeners and gatekeepers running after patients, suddenly bored with their assistant role, bus drivers escorting patient-passengers back to Balmain. Hospital staff were never off duty when it came to escapees: in 1886 escapee Thomas Simpson had the bad luck to run into an ex-attendant in Sydney who recognised him and marched him back to Balmain, and in 1888 patient Josias Keenan was surprised in Campbelltown by two members of staff enjoying a holiday.

10

VOLUNTARY ADMISSIONS

Not everyone was brought to Callan Park forcibly by the police or by concerned relatives or friends. This concept is at odds with the popular myth of nineteenth-century madhouses: as repositories for 'inconvenient' members of society, well or unwell. Madhouses at this time were certainly places of mystery and unease for some, but this attitude persisted thanks largely to the uneducated. For others, they were literally *asylums* – a place of refuge, a place where help might be found and relief gained.

Some men recognised their own symptoms of depression and sought help of their own volition, willingly seeking a place in one of the state's hospitals. Many were disturbed by their own preference for suicide and looked for medical protection from themselves. Sometimes they 'surrendered themselves' to the police or took themselves directly to Reception House or their closest hospital. This 'self' or voluntary admission was not particularly common, and such patients were normally labelled as such in their notes. Such understanding of oneself was regarded as a positive element of mental illness and generally denoted a patient not only *willing* to get better but one who would do so at speed. Some men who arrived at Callan Park were such patients – but this did not by any means preclude them from also being escapees or difficult to manage inmates.

The hospitality and kindness with which such sufferers were treated at Callan Park also opened up Manning's institutions to a small degree of fraud: not every voluntary patient was actually unwell enough to require help. Perhaps the hot baths and regular meals were a little too tempting for some.

William Dwyer,[1] one of Callan Park's early patients, was a carpenter from Sydney. He had a dark complexion with grey eyes and beard, and was of middle height. In 1879 he took himself off to the Central Police Office. Being 'weak ... and shaky' he declared himself of 'unsound mind' and was taken without argument to Reception House. On the first and second day he was the same: tremulous and nervous – but on the third, miraculously, he was much better. He was eating and sleeping well. Despite this, on 19 September 1879, he was taken to Gladesville for treatment. The doctors of the overcrowded hospital, in the throes of transporting the four groups of twelve over to Callan Park to relieve the excessive numbers they were treating, admitted that he was not completely well but 'it was thought advisable to give him a trial' and discharged him after a brief stay there. Like so many, with his newfound freedom Dwyer immediately commenced drinking and 'became very much excited, rambling and incoherent of speech and had delusions that people in fantastic dresses urged him to desperation'. At least, that is what he came to report to police and doctors during his readmission to Reception House a few weeks later. He added that he had attempted to hang himself, complained that he had a hole in his head and had eventually tried to drown himself – and only stopped because he thought he saw a vision in the water. He *told* the Water Police he was insane, they believed him, and he was delivered to Reception House once more. And again, the thirty-year-old followed the same pattern: restless for a couple of days, and then fantastically recovered. This time he was sent not to Gladesville but to Callan Park.

When he arrived at Garryowen he was first installed in Ward One to be observed and classified. He was noted as being well-nourished and clean with no injuries. This was highly unusual for an incoming patient to New South Wales' asylums. Many men, and particularly those who came to hospital via the police, had suffered through either homelessness or violence, and as a result their bodily condition was much below par. But Dwyer was apparently quite well. His pulse was measured at seventy-two, also a reasonable rate for a well man. It was decided that Dwyer was suffering from a delusional type of melancholia, based on the visions he described, and that the duration of his symptoms had been for between three and four years. The doctors at

Callan Park diagnosed sunstroke as the reason for this mental disquiet, in view of his job as a carpenter. But they were intrigued by this man. He was well cared for apparently, and the staff at Callan Park noted with curiosity Dwyer's odd – and convenient – loss of memory when questioned about his past. Mystified, particularly given the two recent attempts to take his own life he had described, it was noted that he did not 'give expression' to any of his *reported* delusions and instead was 'quiet and orderly and industrious'. Such behaviour was unusual – for most patients their first month or so saw an extreme reaction to their new environment. Instead, he took food well and slept well at night. During the day he assisted the carpenter. In short, Dwyer was the perfect patient. It was almost as if he was *enjoying* himself. He lived it up in the hospital, enjoying the meals and attention. At Garryowen for five months, Dwyer was eventually discharged as 'well' in September 1880.

Unhappy at his freedom, between the end of 1880 and September 1881, Dwyer was admitted to Parramatta Hospital for the Insane, Gladesville Hospital and then to Callan Park once more. When he arrived back in Balmain, the Callan Park staff were suspicious. They wrote, 'He is at present in good general health and, as on his last admission, immediately on his arrival at hospital became well and industrious and shows very little sign of insanity'. They did, however, acknowledge his nervousness and propensity to look on the dark side, but this was hardly a reason to require time in an asylum. Dwyer was put under close scrutiny and was perhaps even questioned. Preferring the hospital to the world outside, Dwyer came clean, adding: he could not 'trust himself' outside the bounds of Manning's hospitals. He was an alcoholic, he said, which led to delusions and a preference for suicide. He also really just liked living in the hospital.

Thus Callan Park was presented with a difficult patient to manage. Dwyer was a man in no need of medical assistance: he was sane and able to work, but unable to care for himself if he left the hospital as discharged. Technically this latter aspect – his inability to keep up regular employment to allow him to live well – was reason enough to keep him in care at Callan Park. Dwyer was not discharged; instead, it was decided that he would be tolerated. He was put to work with the carpenter and occasionally let out for the day to build up his independence and resilience with a view, presumably, to his ultimate discharge somewhere in the future when he might be convinced that a life outside the asylum walls was worth living.

Three months into his stay at Callan Park, he was given a day pass and went to Town. Day passes indicated a patient's trustworthiness and also his closeness to discharge; such freedom was used as a test of independence. Perturbed by this, Dwyer wanted to ensure that he was viewed as a patient still in need of medical care. Perhaps to solidly cement in the staff's minds this need for help, or because he actually was an addict, Dwyer promptly went drinking. He was arrested by the police for his bad public behaviour and was subjected to seven days in gaol. Perhaps to allay the response of the hospital's staff, Dwyer's symptoms conveniently worsened upon his return to Balmain. He did not work, for one. For another, he was weak and nervous. Third, he now complained of slight fainting fits, which he hinted might be a sign of his developing epilepsy. But the staff were not so easily fooled: soon Dwyer was working again, happy and content and without any of his fainting attacks. Blaxland's staff finally acknowledged that Dwyer *wanted* to be, and *would* be, a patient for life: 'there is no doubt if discharged he would drink and become as bad as ever'. It is unclear why intemperance was not assumed the cause of his mental health issues.

Dwyer was safe: he had what he wanted – and was classified as a chronic patient who could not be relied upon to look after himself if discharged. But in April 1882 he began acting outside the bounds of his clever brand of lunacy. Either suddenly complacent in terms of his position at the hospital or beginning to demonstrate a lack of logic which was perhaps consistent with a much deeper insanity, he decided to escape. He had been working in the carpentry shop with 'considerable liberty' for some months when Blaxland allowed him permission to accompany the carpenter to Town. He duly did this and gave no one any disquiet. He returned at approximately 4pm and was then sequestered to a job in the medical superintendent's house[2] but was missed at dinner and then tea time due to his escape. The following day the carpenter declared that his glazier's diamond[3] was missing, and the absent Dwyer was accused of the theft. On the third day Dwyer was arrested, drunk, and an attendant went to fetch him from the Central Police Court. On arriving at Callan Park, Dwyer denied all knowledge of the diamond tool.

Such an instance put Blaxland's staff on their guard. Dwyer was being humoured in his place in the hospital, and suspicions about his motives returned. It was with a marked surprise that an actual epileptic fit was recorded in Dwyer's notes two months later: 'Yesterday patient had a marked but not severe epileptic seizure, he felt faint and sat down in a chair at the same time crying out, he grasped an attendant by the hand who distinctly felt it twitch and also saw his mouth slightly convulsed ...' Dwyer became officially epileptic, a patient with a *bona fide* need for treatment at Callan Park, and *petit mal* was added to his list of ailments. It was almost as if he was getting worse by *being* at Callan Park. For three months he recuperated and in the following year was given a three month leave of absence during which his sister cared for him. Blaxland was enormously willing for patients to take up offers of leaves of absence. In 1881 he bemoaned the lack of patients who used this facility:

> *It is to be regretted that friends of patients do not avail themselves more frequently of this system* [leave of absence], *for by it they are enabled to judge if the patient can be managed at home, and in the event of return to hospital being necessary they are spared any fresh expense and the patient any fresh exposure. The change of air and scene is greatly beneficial to some patients, and the knowledge that they may be returned to hospital is a useful form of discipline which calls for the effort of self-control and greatly aids restoration to mental health. They are frequently able also to do some work, and so lessen the cost of their maintenance.*[4]

Two months into his stay with his sister, Dwyer was sent to Reception House on remand. He had been discovered by the police naked and excited, roaming the streets. Manning had to intercede and insisted Dwyer be returned immediately to Callan Park.

Dwyer's sanity did not improve: in October 1883 during a picnic he was allowed a glass of beer. Being a convalescent patient, he was allowed to be around the grounds until 8pm that night but he did not return after the festivities. Blaxland did not blame anyone: Dwyer's hunger for beer had led him to escape and seek more. It was not until eight days later that a telegram arrived at Callan Park saying that Dwyer had given himself up to the Parramatta police. When he was returned, Dwyer said that:

> *he had several glasses of beer during the day he was at the picnic and scarcely knew what he was doing till he got clear of the place* [Callan Park], *he then went on and led a miserable life for a week, fancying that every footstep he heard was that of someone after him, he did a little work and on Thursday (25th) started to walk back from Blacktown but feeling miserable at Parramatta he gave himself up to the police. He states that he did not drink during the time he was away and did not look as if he had been on his return.*

Dwyer could not restrain himself: a year later he disappeared again, on Christmas Day. In January 1885, unable to be found within twenty-eight days, Dwyer was discharged from Callan Park's books.

Of course, Dwyer obliged his own instincts in self-preservation and returned to hospital again. By 1891 Callan Park staff were used to this yo-yoing escapee: 'this patient when convalescent prefers leaving the institution [by escape] ... to being discharged in the ordinary manner'.

But not every voluntary patient was like fickle and fair-weather Dwyer. Some were rather more desperate for help. Charles Hampden Merritt,[5] the man who discovered Morton's knife concealed in the earth pit in 1883, was one such man. At only twenty-three when he first sought help, Merritt came to spend his lifetime in care. In 1879 he decided to commit himself into the care of Manning's hospitals. Merritt was epileptic and suffering additionally from dementia. His fits were preceded by a 'peculiar feeling in the head in which he described a lost feeling' and his memory was greatly impaired. He told medical staff that he had been afraid of seeking help, since this would mean leaving home and that he might 'lose himself' as a consequence. There is no record of Merritt at Reception House, and it is possible that he merely arrived at Gladesville Hospital begging for help. Seven months later he was transferred to Callan Park.

Callan Park agreed that he was exhibiting the classic symptoms of epilepsy but were disturbed by the letters he wrote. While sometimes obstinate and irritable, Merritt was largely submissive and manageable: except in his letter writing. In notes to friends and family he was recorded as having been sustainedly angry, complaining constantly of his ill-treatment and abuse at the hospital. Unlike George Morton, whose letters were kept as evidence of his insanity for Whitehall, none of Merritt's confiscated letters survive today.

Merritt's early days in Balmain were characterised by frequent mild attacks of epilepsy. In 1881 Merritt and William Andrews,[6] both patients of Ward Two, began to clash. Andrews was a labourer from Orange and had first become registered at Gladesville in 1877. He was a sufferer of mania brought about by his epilepsy, and when he first arrived at hospital came with a broken nose, the result of a bout of excited activity. Four years previously he had been gaoled for selling his employer's cattle while in a drunken state. His time in gaol had exacerbated a pre-existing propensity for fits, and in the previous eighteen months had developed the disease. He was anything but a voluntary patient. During his initial treatment he was 'restless and unsteady and childish' which was characteristic of his recovery from 'epileptic paroxysm[s]'. Like Merritt, Andrews suffered from infrequent fits but was otherwise quite content working in the wood yard and the gardens, planting the new flower beds around the Kirkbride complex. Also similar to Merritt, Andrews was convinced he was being persecuted and maltreated, particularly by poison-happy relatives, and was as a result often violent. Gladesville called him 'imprudent and abusive' and a man who was often confined to his single room for his own and others' sakes. He also thought that he was Jesus, but confused staff by both singing hymns and blaspheming. Both men were young and strong: Williams not only cut wood but broke down doors in Garryowen and was perhaps one of those who was responsible for the breaking of the glass windows in the weatherboard extension beside

Garryowen. In 1880 Andrews suffered a severe fit which left his right arm paralysed, his face 'fallen' and his speech badly affected. Suddenly Andrews was unable to act on his violent inclinations.

Merritt thus fought with a handicapped foe and both were secluded for their behaviour at various times. Andrews was transferred to Rydalmere in 1893, his fits often leading to severe falls and head injuries; Merritt left Callan Park for Parramatta in 1891. Like Andrews, Merritt was described as becoming ever more 'demented' as he neared middle age. He was not happy being kept in care anymore, and persisted at Parramatta in escape attempts, making knives out of bits of tin he found. A year later, after a debilitating injury to his hip, the product of a fall, he 'sank and died'.

Not every voluntary patient was young and angry however, and not all of them arrived at the hospital initially of their own free will, perhaps frightened by what might lie beyond the gates of an asylum. George Merry[7] was one such man and was initially brought to Manning's institution against his own inclination. Merry, a small, vulnerable man, arrived in Sydney in 1853 on board the *Great Britain*, the same ship Frederick Legard also took at one point in his many trips between Australia and England. For the next twenty years Merry built up a small fortune via the gold fields of Australia which amounted at his death to £723. In 1873 however, he became unwell. At the same time a notice was placed in the *Police Gazette* and entitled 'Missing Friends'.[8] Information regarding Merry was requested by the Inspector General of Police; he had not been responding to letters from his family and friends.

Three years later, with his pockets full of more than £22 cash, Merry, described as a 'miner', was brought to Reception House from the Central Police Office. The forty-eight-year-old refused all food and was fitted with a straightjacket, presumably to protect him from himself. Low spirited and convinced terrible calamities were about to befall him, but without any actual delusions, Merry was suffering from melancholia which rose and fell with his bodily health. He was taken to Gladesville where his symptoms improved with rest, shelter and food; soon he was transferred to the branch establishment at Callan Park as one of the first forty-four. Intelligent and manageable, particularly as he was 'a strict abstainer from alcohol and [would] not take any stimulant', he was an ideal first patient at Garryowen and it was noted in is file that he took 'a great interest in the institution'. There he was free from 'melancholic attacks' for some time and found great industry in the 'animals, dogs and other things'. Merry was therefore one of the patients who initiated the menagerie at Callan Park which was to grow to hold wallabies, kangaroos and flying squirrels, and was probably witness to, and affected by, Legard's murder of one of the pets in 1879. Merry's progress while caring for the animals was so good that he was soon discharged in February 1880 as 'recovered'. He was one of Callan Park's first successes.

Merry was well again. He had money to support himself and he used this to travel to Melbourne to make a fresh start. For some time he supported himself in Victoria, but eventually returned to Sydney. Increasingly depressed, he found he 'could not get on in the world' due to his symptoms. In May 1880, tearful and plagued by morbid thoughts, he 'returned to the hospital of his own accord'. Staff at Callan Park agreed with this course of action, adding to his notes that 'hospital is ... the best place for him'. Silent and reserved, but trustworthy, Merry worked in the store alongside Legard, and continued to look after the animals and poultry on the farm. His time at Callan Park was idyllic. He was safe and happy, and only disturbed when he considered the idea of ever being sent away: '[he] bursts into tears at the idea of being sent away from hospital'. By 1890, during the census of Callan Park in which many chronic patients were moved to Parramatta and Rydalmere, Merry was described as 'demand[ing] his release then beg[ging] with tears to be kept safe'. At this point he was rather thin and feeble. He stayed at Callan Park until his death in 1895 of phthisis, a wasting disease of a type with tuberculosis.

Merry was one of a very few patients of Callan Park who died with any kind of money to his name. Even more unusually, he had a will. After his death James Scott Patterson, a legal manager of various mines in Australia, placed a notice in the *Government Gazette*[9] announcing Merry's decease and calling for creditors to contact his solicitor to make their claims upon his estate. Merry's wealth was entirely in cash, not in land or equipment, with

£611 in the control of the master-in-lunacy. Merry had no wife or children, or indeed any recorded family living in Australia.

While Merry sought help from Callan Park to combat his depression, Samuel Wade[10] went to the Central Police Office for protection against himself in 1878. Desperate and deluded, his 'wild and strange manner of speaking' quickly convinced the officers of his need for medical attention. While in their custody he cut his own throat but had no memory of the act the next day. At Reception House more evidence of his insanity came to light when he fell during a fit. Wade's forehead, heavily scared, was proof of his ongoing epilepsy: he had been hitting his head for thirty-five of his thirty-nine years of life.

Wade had been proactive, asking for help in dealing with his insanity: he was treated at Reception House and then transferred to Gladesville, where he thought he would be safe. Between October 1878 and September 1879 he had many fits, which were followed by 'mental dullness and irresponsibility'. Two weeks before his transfer to Callan Park he attempted to hang himself with his comforter in the recreation paddock. Wade had asked for help, but Staff found that, short of allocating him a personal attendant, they could not always supervise him against himself.

Callan Park was told that Wade required 'watching and attention' and his mother, half a world away in Pudsey in England, was informed by letter of her son's removal to Balmain. But again, staffing meant that Wade could not have constant supervision. In 1880 he interrupted a calm walk around the hospital grounds by suddenly rushing into the water, after having thrown aside his coat. The water lapping around his waist, Wade stopped and attendant Sherack, seeing him, caught up and walked him back to shore. At other times Wade would write letters to God and 'complain[ed] ... of not receiving any reply' and said that he received messages from 'him that's above' from 'the 'ead office'. In 1883 he was informed that such letters were not sent and was abusive in response. He was often secluded for throwing stones and breaking down the door of his room. When suicidal however, Wade received the attention he had begged for at the police station and of the hospital staff. The staff were vigilant in this and to their credit he was never successful in ending his own life. He was transferred to Rydalmere in 1893 and was eventually buried near the gates at Rookwood cemetery.

Voluntary patients were not common in Manning's institutions, and from their behaviour it would not have been at all clear that they had begged for protection from themselves before arriving at Callan Park. Even though these men were not always manageable by any means, they were provided nonetheless with care, food and shelter by Blaxland and his staff. They were welcomed back after escapes, and their lives were saved by attendants on more than one occasion. It cannot be doubted that Callan Park was a safe and prosperous place to be – or why else return? Why else cry at the thought of being made to leave? These are happy stories, of men who found peace and contentment, even if it was only temporary – but the happiest of all were those men who found permanent cure after their time in Blaxland's hospital and who were discharged, never to return. These men moved on in their lives, happy in the knowledge that they were 'fixed' and Callan Park not a part of their future.

11

RECOVERED

Contrary to the unfounded beliefs of many, the ultimate goal of every doctor in all of Manning's institutions, including Callan Park, was to make each patient 'fit for discharge' due to their 'cure'. Being 'fit for discharge' carried many implications: that the patient's disease – be it mania, melancholia or dementia – was at an end; that the patient could 'get on' in the world and look after himself as any other person might; and that he was unlikely to relapse and cause harm to another person. Manning's aim was for his institutions to be places of high turnover, where patients were treated and then discharged, if possible, and not 'cemeteries'[1] for the mentally ill. Of course, many patients would never get to this point, and would spend the rest of their lives in care as 'chronic patients'. Some who were 'discharged as cured', like George Merry and William Dwyer, in his early association with Gladesville and Callan Park, found themselves back again either through their own volition or via the heavy hand of the police. There were success stories, however: some patients who were said to be cured did not ever return to Manning's asylum system.

Joshua Fitzpatrick[2] was one of these men who was helped by Manning's doctors and found a cure to his mental illness. Fitzpatrick was born in 1859 in Victoria. For reasons which are lost to history, his parents had him declared a ward of the state and sailed for New Zealand where they set up home without their son. Joshua's mother suffered from melancholia and it is possible that her illness required a change of scene. Whatever the reason, Fitzpatrick was brought up in care, possibly through the Marist Brotherhood, but maintained some contact with his own family. As a young adult he trained as a saddler and also became a teacher at the Marist school in Sydney. At this time, and possibly the reason for his parental desertion, he was described as a boy of 'weak intellect'.[3]

One day in 1877, when he was eighteen, Fitzpatrick left the Marist school where he was working. He told his colleagues there that he was going to take a steamer to New Zealand to stay with his parents. He packed his box and bid them goodbye. The following day, the Marist Brothers were contacted by a Sydney pawnbroker, Mr Hayes, who said that Fitzpatrick's case had been found abandoned and open in Lower Fort Street. Upon checking the shipping timetables, it was quickly realised that no ship had left for New Zealand on the day Fitzpatrick had said goodbye. He was missing and fears for his safety were raised.[4] A notice was placed in the *Police Gazette* under the title 'Missing Friends': anyone who had seen the mid-height teenager with dark, short hair and a dark complexion, was asked to contact the Inspector General of Police.

Reception House, via Manning, contacted the Inspector General of Police: they had Fitzpatrick. Wondering the streets for four and a half days, the teenager had been picked up and delivered to Reception House in a quiet but confused state. On the second day of his stay there he had become suddenly aggressive and violent and could only be managed by the application of a straightjacket. On the third day he was subdued and quiet once more. On the fourth he was transferred to Gladesville Hospital for the Insane.

At Gladesville Fitzpatrick was called poor in bodily health, and stubborn. Revolted by his lack of liberty, he refused to take the medicine which was prescribed for him and the staff were forced to administer this through his nose instead. Obstinate and rude, Fitzpatrick was diagnosed with low intellect and a delusional form of melancholia. He attempted escape, indicating a deep unhappiness at his confinement. In December 1879 he was transferred out to Callan Park along with the likes of Chan Long and Samuel Payne. Unlike many of the other patients who were transferred out simply to relieve the overcrowding at Gladesville, Fitzpatrick was *required* to leave. The reason was simple: in October he had almost been 'successful in planning and carrying out by means of another patient the murder of the Medical Superintendent'. This little gem of a warning was amended to the bottom of the notes which accompanied Fitzpatrick on his transfer to Callan Park, and written in a tiny and almost illegible script. The attempted killing of staff was not unheard of in these hospitals: George Morton told Blaxland that he had wanted his 'heart's blood' and had thus stolen a knife; attendant Perryman was almost killed in 1894 at the farm. Fitzpatrick was worryingly clever, something which was echoed repeatedly in his notes where he was described as 'delight[ing] in making mischief amongst his fellow patients'. In his attempted murder of the doctor he had convinced fellow patient Wilkie to attack as the doctor inspected the wards and work buildings. Wilkie played his part well and was nearly successful: 'Wilkie made a desperate attack upon the Med[ical Sup[erin]t[endant] with a piece of skirting iron and was only frustrated by the activity ... of an Officer (William Betts). The Med[ical] Sup[erin]t[endant] was not injured'. Manning decided that Fitzpatrick needed a change of scene to aid in his recuperation, and so included him in the fourth group of twelve to move to Callan Park.

Callan Park decided that Fitzpatrick's insanity was hereditary, perhaps gaining this information from Fitzpatrick himself, or from visiting Marist Brothers. His mother and sister were both sufferers of what we would today know as depression. Fitzpatrick was already showing signs of distress at Reception House and Gladesville. Now launched into the unfamiliar surroundings of Balmain, and rejoined with patients like Parcelli whom he had previously known at Gladesville, and fought with, Fitzpatrick became worse. He developed hallucinations of hearing, where the voices told him, day and night, that his character was being damaged by 'people writing to the newspapers about him'. He continued to be mischievous and 'foul-tongued' to both staff and patients. He went straight to Ward Two, and into one of the single rooms there 'to prevent [his] escape'.

But this single room did not work: within two months Fitzpatrick had demonstrated his aptitude for escape once more. In late December 1879, after lights were off and patients expected to be sleeping, he managed to get over the roof of Garryowen and escape. It still being light at 7.45pm, he was seen and run down. He was redeposited in his room, but got out again, this time through the door of the ward, at 10pm. Again he was taken by staff. For the next three nights his hands were encased in muffs to prevent any further nocturnal mischief. Fitzpatrick's desire to be gone from Balmain was centred partly on Manning and his colleagues, of whom he seems to have been genuinely terrified. Not only did he try to have Gladesville's superintendent killed, but his delusions also focused on staff. He was convinced that Parkes and Manning, as cronies of the government, were trying to keep him 'out of £30,000', and that someone named 'Joseph' – possibly his father – 'tried to "do for him" with "slow poison"'.

Fitzpatrick presented the same dilemma to Manning and Blaxland as Parcelli did: the facilities at Garryowen could not contain violent patients prone to escape. Fitzpatrick had been moved from Gladesville to separate him from Wilkie and to provide a means of a change of scene to aid in his cure. In early 1880 there was only one other place patients could be sent to: Parramatta.

Gloomy, prison-like Parramatta held both free and criminal lunatics. Manning still did not like the place as in any way conducive to cure or even successful therapy but it was the only other alternative for Fitzpatrick. The patient was transferred with notes describing him as quiet but 'requir[ing of] close watching to prevent his escape'.

Staff at Parramatta were impressed with his 'excellent health' but saddened by his lack of mental progress. They noted, in concurrence with past events, that he 'speaks disrespectfully of medical officers' but, and mimicking the discovery no doubt positively harnessed by the Marist Brothers, he was 'manageable when reasoned with and confidence placed in him'. In three months, rapid progress was made: Fitzpatrick was 'No trouble. He works well, and is healthy'. In May he was still improving and devoting himself to painting. In June, still working with the painter, and having made 'considerable mental improvement', Fitzpatrick began to 'talk about his discharge'.

Fitzpatrick was clever and stubborn: he felt well again and wanted liberation. He had been transferred to Ward Three, a sign of his convalescence and closeness to discharge, but he was anxious to be free. He seized his opportunity somewhat prematurely: one night in July 1880 he was in the billiards room with an attendant who was called away to assist another patient. Suddenly alone and desperate to be out of hospital, Fitzpatrick stole out into the yard of his ward – and to his delight saw that the gate of Ward Two, his old ward, had been erroneously left open. Nimble, Fitzpatrick went through it and disappeared into the night. Eight days later he was still not returned.

A notice was posted in the *Police Gazette* on 14 July:[5]

> *Escaped Lunatic*
> *Parramatta – Escaped, about 8pm on the 5th instant, from the Parramatta Lunatic Asylum, Joshua Fitzpatrick. He is about 25 years of age, 5 feet 8 inches high, medium build, fair complexion, black hair, no whiskers, small black moustache; dressed in brown tweed sac coat, gray tweed trousers, lace-up boots, brown felt hat, white shirt, and blue and white necktie.*

Fitzpatrick was having a miserable time. He was homeless and starving and had been forced to visit the soup kitchen to support himself. During this time of 'self-effected liberty', as the Parramatta staff chose to call it, he had had one goal: to present the facts of his situation to several lawyers in the hope that they could win for him a legal liberty. Going about this in Sydney Fitzpatrick eventually ran into an attendant of his old hospital, Callan Park, who insisted that he return to Balmain with him. From there, he was transferred safely back to Parramatta.

The staff at Parramatta punished him for his truancy and stopped him from 'work[ing] as he used to' for fear of him slipping out again. But in another month he was not troublesome any more. By November his delusions were 'less obvious' and he was trusted to work again with the painter. Unbelievably in December 1880 he was discharged as cured.

In 1877 Fitzpatrick had been interrupted by a sudden turn on his way to see his parents. The interval had been a long one – three years of care under Manning's wing – but he determined to persevere with his original plans. Fitzpatrick left New South Wales and sailed for New Zealand. He lived quietly and as a result did not make a heavy footprint in the historical record. But in the 1890 New Zealand Electoral Roll there is a James Joshua Fitzpatrick, a saddler, living in Clyde on the South Island, just North-West of Dunnedin. He died in New Zealand in Raurimu, on the North Island, in 1925.

Fitzpatrick had proved himself well enough for discharge but only by escaping, conducting some unsuccessful discussions with lawyers, and then proving his mental wellness after the fact. James McMahon had a similar end goal in mind but conducted himself rather differently and in a far less convoluted manner.

James, or sometimes John, McMahon[6] was a man who had a terrible temper. When he had been twenty-five, in the 1860s, he had suffered a terrible head injury. Over the following years he had become increasingly restless and flighty. In addition, he became possessed of the idea that his family was 'unfairly' using him and as a result became increasingly suspicious of his parents. On a number of occasions he threatened them in what he thought was self-defence. As a labourer in Kiama he assaulted one of his colleagues and followed another with the intention of shooting him. Finally, he began to speak to his family of his desire to commit suicide.

At Reception House, where he was admitted in 1878, he was quiet and orderly by day and night. He was the same at Gladesville, working well in the grounds and giving no trouble. In 1879 when he was moved to Callan Park, a few years before the Kirkbride Complex's final completion, he was described as having a 'weak silly expression' along with a terrible temper that 'when roused might be uncontrollable'. He was, though, 'very quiet, well conducted and willing to make himself useful'. Like Frederick Legard, much his senior, McMahon was also labelled as 'an odd, peculiar' man. But there was nothing at Callan Park to trigger that uncontrollable temper of his, no infuriating colleagues or meddling family members, and McMahon found himself quickly recovering. For years he was contained and treated with respect and dignity, and he continued to improve. He was allowed 'considerable liberty' around the grounds of the hospital, something which might have earned him the jealousy of patients like Fitzpatrick. He was even trusted to work at the far reaches of the park, maintaining the cottages there.

In July 1882 McMahon made his most significant ploy to end his time in care. He designed a rather attractive petition for his own release, decorated with ornate lettering. He asked the various contractors on site, who were building the Kirkbride Complex, and the artisans at Garryowen, to sign it. Soon after, he presented it to Blaxland:

> *WE THE CONTRACTORS ENGINEERS AND ARTISANS OF CALLAN PARK MAGNUM OPUS ASYLUM*
> *Through long and careful scrutiny along with numerous interviews, together with over two years close observation we believe James McMahon an inmate now in Callan Park Madhouse to be perfectly sane in every point of view and we one and all write in righteously demanding his release, he being held captive in madhouses for over four years which we think to be an outrage on the Justice and a great national disgrace. The said James McMahon being in the bloom of lief* [sic] *and health and a first class all round workman, as well as being charitable*[ly] *disposed, a poet and an intelligent member of society.*

It was signed by a total of four men whom he worked with around the grounds of the asylum. Blaxland initialled it under the descriptor 'Specimen of a testimonial drawn up by James McMahon', dated it, and glued it into McMahon's pages in the *Medical Case Books*.

For those who have read stories from England at this time – Charles Reade's *Hard Cash,* Wilkie Collins' *Woman in White* – this would seem a plan unlikely to work. But the popular belief concerning the difficulty of discharging oneself from an insane hospital once arrived, which was the focus of numerous fictions at the time, did not apply to Manning's hospitals. These were state run institutions: if a patient was well, there was no reason to keep his bed from someone else who needed it. Blaxland and Manning received no 'back-handers' for keeping certain men within their walls. The procedures for complaints were transparent. Petitions for 'release' fell not on deaf ears but were attended to and sometimes acted upon. In England, attempting to withdraw oneself, once committed, from a private asylum was almost impossible, even with the Lord Chancellor's official visitors. Indeed, in England a group named the Alleged Lunatics' Friend Society (ALFS), begun by several including John Perceval, operated with the specific function of advocating for men and women *alleged* to be mad, who had found little help within the existing system. The ALFS represented and assisted such 'prisoners' by petitioning MPs and alerting the media to examples of wrongful confinement.

But the situation was not so dire, the stakes not so high, for common labourers in New South Wales' public asylums. McMahon was discharged by Blaxland to the care of a friend, as cured as anyone with an untreated head injury could ever be. He was readmitted for a short time a couple of decades later, but otherwise kept free of care for the rest of his life. Such was the design of Manning, who was a firm believer in the power of family care in the aiding of the recovery of the insane. He wrote in 1868[7] that 'Every effort should be made to induce families to receive back again their insane members'. Further, that, 'There is no reason why the patient should not return to his home, where he can be fed, lodged, clothed, and watched over, by those near and dear to him, provided an allowance for his support is made to his family, equal to, or even smaller than, that which he costs in the asylum itself'.[8]

Some patients, of course, played upon this keen sense of family support in Manning's vision of care. Henry Jones, for example, tried to use it to effect his removal from Callan Park, when he was actually still very ill. But faking recovery was something that staff were constantly on the alert to, and not so easily fooled.

Henry Jones[9] was to blame for his own degeneracy and insanity. A bank clerk for his career, first in England and later working for the Bank of New South Wales, he was also an alcoholic. His intemperance had stirred a flicker of dementia in his mind and by 1877, when his wife took him to Gladesville Hospital, he was severely demented and in dire need of medical help. He was unable to work at this time. Upon his removal to hospital he spoke the most 'random and inconsequent statements especially as to dates and places, was extremely nervous and in a weak condition of general health'.

He was at Gladesville for a year and a half before being named as one of the first forty-four and was installed at Garryowen with Legard and Merry. Upon his arrival the sixty-one-year-old was described as being in the advanced stages of dementia, with a severe loss of memory. With relief, it was recorded that he was cleanly and keen to work in the wood yard. Like Legard he was drafted in to assist in the office on the top floor of Garryowen and also went 'frequently to Mr Whitling', the clerk and deputy superintendent of Callan Park. How much help he was in administration is unclear since he could only write 'a little and connected letters but it [was] very doubtful if his faculties [were] sufficiently restored to enable him to gain a livelihood'. It was therefore more likely that his visits were part of his therapy – not designed to assist in Manning's institutions, but to help with his memory loss and self-esteem.

Through 1879 Jones continued to be cheerful and was in good health; he even made some mental improvement. In December, as a mark of his increasing health, he was allowed a leave of absence to visit his son in Sydney. Why Manning and Scholes held such faith in leaves of absence when they so often went wrong – ending in arrest or temporary escape – is a mystery. Such freedom was too much for Jones: he did not return at the appointed time, due to his arrest for public drunkenness. One wonders where his son was at this point. Whatever the events of the day, Jones was blacklisted for future leaves of absence by Scholes. As a result, it was entered in his notes that discharge would be probably impossible for Jones, as he could not be trusted for a 'single day'.

Surely this mistrust was communicated to Jones because he was well behaved for some time after, working quietly in the grounds and office. In April 1880 he was given another chance. Jones conducted himself with decorum this time and came back to the hospital at the appointed hour, and without the stench of liquor on his breath. Why this good behaviour, and where he had actually been for the day, was only discovered later. While Scholes was basking in optimism for his patient after this seeming success, a letter arrived at Callan Park for Manning. It was from a Dr Moffett a 'physician and surgeon', of 3 Lyon's Terrace in Sydney. It read:

> *I have known Mr Henry Jones for over 20 years in connection with the London Chardered* [sic] *Bank and the Bank of New South Wales, as his Medical adviser, attending on himself and wife – and I have never seen during my attendance upon him any symptoms of insanity – I have lost sight of him for the last three years or there about, but to today and saw him again and believe him to be perfectly sane.*

Manning was flabbergasted – outraged – that one of his patients had been so bold as to find a tame physician to write him what was essentially a contrary diagnosis. The Inspector General of the Insane fired a letter back to Moffett, whose reply was pasted into Jones' *Medical Case Book* pages as a record of the patient's audacity and desperation of escape.

> *My Dear Dr Manning,*
> *I received yours of yesterday, concerning a certificate given by me to Mr Henry Jones – who called upon me on the 11th instant, being on old patient of over 20 years and not having seen him for some years past, I was greatly surprised to find that he had been a patient at Gladesville and Callan Pk for the last three years, he spoke so rationally and pleaded so earnestly for a certificate, which he said would procure his release, that I was induced to give him the certificate to which you allude, not for one moment reflecting on Dr Scholes or yourself, as I thought his release or retention rested entirely with you – the particulars of his case which you have given, are for the most part new to me, and had I known them, I would most certainly have refused the certificate ...* [I see] *Now that he is not capable of taking care of himself or conducting any business except under strong control I shall feel much obliged if you will make my apology to Dr Scholes, and accept the same yourself for*

this unwarranted interference with your respective duties and believe me

Very truthfully yours,
A Moffett

Sense prevailed and Moffett was made to retract his ill-advised certificate of sanity. Six months later Jones was still 'very much impaired' but was still able to write. Manning and Scholes doubted however his ability to look after himself and also the keenness of his family to look after him. As a result, he was given the run of the park and worked happily until his death in 1903.

Henry Jones had tried his damnedest to secure his liberation, but it was not to be. Manning, Scholes and Blaxland were not so easily fooled by their patients. Their jobs were to care for these insane men, even battle with them over their own wellbeing, and protect the public which lived beyond the walls of the asylum. Fitzpatrick and McMahon were successes to be celebrated: they had means to make a living and the mental health to ensure their uninterrupted independence. Jones had tried to fake this, and as a result retained his place amongst the swelling ranks of Callan Park's inmates. Many of the original patients of Manning's Balmain hospital were in the same boat as Jones. They might not have run to a tame and friendly doctor, but they were patients for life like him: sometimes dangerous but always unable to care for themselves in the world outside.

12

CHRONIC PATIENTS

Most patients in Manning's institutions were chronic patients. Most frequently brought into Callan Park by the police, these men were labelled permanently unfit for discharge. The overwhelming majority of the patients described in this book were chronic since staff at Callan Park did not trust them to look after themselves beyond the walls of the hospital. The likelihood of their injuring themselves or some other member of the public was high, given their often-maniacal dispositions and physical strength. They often had no family or friends who might act as a support during their release back into the community, and so were kept in the hospital – given care, food and shelter. As a result, they often lived long lives. The variety of work and amusements on offer suggests that these were happy lives.

For many years after its inception Callan Park was the main receiving hospital for the Sydney metropolitan district. As a result it was in a unique position: most of Sydney's insane passed through its wards, normally at the beginning of their treatment. Some stayed for the rest of their care, but other hospitals such as Parramatta, Rydalmere and Kenmore began more and more to take the chronic patients. By the turn of the century Callan Park was more a centre for acute therapy, with its patients either being discharged as cured after a brief stint there or transferred out to one of the hospitals for the chronically insane.

As Sydney's main receiving hospital, Callan Park was also the hospital which was most often lumbered with foreign patients 'direct from the ships in which they arrived in the Colony, or immediately after landing'.[1] These were often chronic patients, whose passage to New South Wales had been bought by relatives usually from Britain, neighbouring colonies and the South Sea Islands[2] with the wish that they might be free of the care of their insane family member. Of course, some were merely accidents: American Josias Keenan[3] had been perfectly well in mind and body when he left his wife and America to travel the world, and eventually ended up in Australia. Intoxicated one night when only newly arrived, he fell and hit his head. For the next twelve years he had moments of memory of his old life, and eventually died of a cerebral haemorrhage at Callan Park.

This is not to say that every new arrival to the colony was insane: indeed, John McDonald Brennan, who arrived in Queensland in July 1874, was anything but mad. But he was trying to escape the insane.

John Brennan's family had a strong hereditary lunacy running through it, with his mother, brother, sister, uncle, aunt and cousin, all living in Glasgow in Scotland, ill with a delusional form of melancholia. The burden which this must have created for the well members of John Brennan's family – particularly on his father and himself – must have been huge. John Brennan was a doctor, having studied medicine in Glasgow where he graduated as a surgeon in 1863. When he was thirty-seven he decided to leave his family and, like Legard and Parcelli, begin a new life on the other side of the world. A year and a half after his arrival in Queensland Dr John Brennan was a registered doctor in New South Wales and he chose, ironically, Balmain as his place of abode and work at the exact time John Keep and his neighbours were petitioning against the new madhouse in their suburb. For some time John Brennan was known as the 'principal doctor'[4] in the locale and enjoyed a wholesome and knowledgeable reputation there.

Dr John Brennan was free: he ran a thriving practice and was no longer responsible for the upkeep of his unwell family. But this respite was only of three years duration: in 1879 his younger brother William[5] sailed on the *Samuel Plimsoll* to join him in Balmain. John Brennan discovered that while on board, his brother had been 'low-spirited'. John Brennan's heart must have sunk – and Manning's too. William Brennan's arrival in New South Wales was exactly what the Inspector General of the Insane was striving to avoid.

The care of such a man ought to be shouldered by the Scottish tax payers, not those in New South Wales. A month into William's residence in Balmain, and literally in the shadow of Callan Park, he was increasingly melancholy and restless by night. He 'fancied people were waiting about to take him away' and was particularly concerned that one of these people was the captain of the *Samuel Plimsoll* who he thought was waiting to kidnap him in a carriage. Echoing his mother and her family, he began to threaten suicide.

John, knowing well the signs of insanity, took his brother to the Water Police Office in October of that year – only three months out from William's arrival. Older brother could not care for younger now. John could manage low spirits and mild delusions, but potential suicide he could not. Installed at Reception House, William was quiet and slept well. Given John's proximity to Callan Park, William was taken there and was admitted outside the four sets of twelve from Gladesville which were occurring at the same time. Upon his arrival, William's symptoms became worse: he would sigh and sob and was increasingly paranoid that he was about to be kidnapped. And while he could give 'a connected account of himself' he began to exhibit religious delusions. The obsessive Catholic told staff that 'he ha[d] lost the graces of God and [could not] recover it and that suicide [was] the only remedy for him'. John Brennan was a devout Catholic, regularly attending mass at St Joseph's Church in Newtown up until his death in 1909 which was recorded in the *Catholic Press*.[6] Like many of his fellow patients, William had turned his religion into a delusion. He feared the wrath of God and thought suicide the only remedy. But William Brennan was not alone in these notions.

Religious delusions flourished at Callan Park, the patients often feeding off each others' frenzied ideas, and hampering their own recovery as a result. William Brennan was partly responsible for some of this. George Morton complained that Brennan had created his, Morton's, delusions, among which were ideas that to drink would drown the Virgin Mary who was inside him. He wrote in a confiscated letter in 1883:

> *I was troubled by religion – and voices. It was all fancy. Caused by the man William Brennan, a Patient, talking religion to me*

especially about fasting & praying which I did not believe in. He said, I would be 'd'-'d' if I ate. This annoyed me; and brought me down very low – He had great influence over me, through being of a religious turn of mind and I tried to fast; but could, or would not, and my conscience brought me down very low; and I ate – What do you think??? ??? ??? ??? He is a scoundrel; and a reprobate – no more! ... I am completely well of weakness, and all the hellish woe caused by Brennan, in me, and got completely well of debility.[7]

But Morton and Brennan were not the only chronic patients affected by religion. Terence McGuire,[8] a man in his thirties like Brennan and who arrived in New South Wales on the same ship but the year before, also suffered from vivid religious hallucinations. When he arrived in Sydney with his brothers in 1878 McGuire was completely well. He and his brothers were assisted immigrants to New South Wales and they travelled to Orange to work. But by November of the same year, though still 'talkative and jovial' McGuire 'fancied that he had come down from Heaven and that Jesus was constantly speaking to him'. In addition, he was under the impression that a priest had robbed him of £4000 and was increasingly obsessed with King Soloman. He would talk incessantly to himself, and was impervious to pain, being about to pluck out all of his facial hair without feeling anything. He was taken to Gladesville and then Callan Park where he lived until his transfer to Parramatta in 1891.

Simon Patrick Holland,[9] one of the first forty-four, was the same. Married with five children, Holland had started life in New South Wales as a police constable. He hailed from Ireland and after a few years as a policeman opened up a hotel. Thin and with a 'cadaverous dark' complexion and 'grizzled hair closely cropped' in 1876 he was taken to Reception House where he was noisy and troublesome. Answering most questions upon arrival at Gladesville with 'I don't know', he spent most of his time praying and worrying over his supposed poisoning. William Brennan was in a hot house of religious delusions where he shared and borrowed from his fellow patients.

While the short distance from his surgery to Garryowen House must have made visiting William quite easy for John Brennan, there were also many issues associated with living so near the asylum. For one, William Brennan – unlike most other escapees but very like Alex Clubb – was highly knowledgeable about his location which made vanishing from care all the easier. In October 1879 Brennan was described as cheerful and working well in the grounds. This, as it turned out, was a rouse to patrol the area and begin a reconnaissance which would end in his escape. In December, attendant James Hain took a working party of patients out to continue building the new recreation grounds. At noon, which was break time, Brennan followed instructions with his fellow inmates, left his tools in the tool house and received his beer in the courtyard of Garryowen. As per normal routine, the patients were separated into groups denoting their ward and those from Ward Two went with outdoor attendant Cheetham by the dispensary and back inside. Cheetham, counting the men back into their weatherboard ward, found one short. An immediate search for Brennan was made – but no trace of him could be found. Brennan had merely retraced his steps and made his way back to the recreation grounds. From there he climbed through a drain which got him outside of the bounds of Garryowen and into the general park. From there, he made his way smartly to his brother's house.

What was most interesting was that his brother hid him for seven days from hospital staff and the police. John Brennan was not married, and never would be: his only family in Australia was William. Perhaps he enjoyed the company. At this time William Brennan was much recovered and recommended himself for discharge by his positivity and wellbeing. On 23 December a constable Ross sighted William Brennan at his brother's house. But John persevered: he kept his brother over Christmas and only brought him back on Boxing Day because staff and the police continued to focus surveillance on his house. John Brennan applied on New Year's Eve for the discharge of his brother into his own care. John Brennan's optimism is saddening. On the same day of his happy application, his brother was secluded with – notably given the nature of his delusions – *Reverend* Legard for assaulting one of the Ward Two attendants. A week later, perhaps unenlightened by hospital staff, his brother took him home.

Five months later, and possibly after a seven-day gaol sentence for public drunkenness, William Brennan was delivered back to Callan Park by his brother. The dawning realisation that his brother was just as ill as the majority of his extended family, must have hit John Brennan hard. Perhaps he had been filled with thoughts of managing William on his own – he *was* a doctor after all – but this was now impossible: Brennan's delusions and suicidal thoughts had returned and he was losing weight again. Callan Park was nonplussed and unsurprised at Brennan's return. Staff comments were clear on the issue: 'mentally he is the same'. Soon Brennan began 'annoying' Legard again, indicating his delusions were in full flight once more. He made 'no mental improvement' but rather was 'sly and takes every opportunity of attempting to escape'. In October he pulled patient John Dye, an old and feeble man, out of bed, and the elderly man flung him down and broke Brennan's left clavicle. This childishness was summed up in Brennan's later comment that the injury 'served me right', and, later, his constant worrying of his bandages. A week after the incident and rather indicative of John Brennan's realisation that his brother would was suffering a chronic form of insanity, the Balmain doctor requested that William be transferred to Gladesville. John Brennan suggested this as a way to curb William's frequent escape attempts. He also added that his 'professional prospects' were being impacted by his lunatic brother. His close proximity to William must have meant frequent visits to the hospital, something which cannot have always been pleasant. Aside from the noise and atmosphere at Garryowen at this time – there were over 100 men there – observation by staff cannot have been easy for John Brennan, almost the sole member of his family untouched by delusions. Manning himself wrote on this phenomenon:

> *The hereditary transmission of insanity is a subject of the most profound interest, both from a medical and social standpoint, and to a medical superintendent of a hospital for the insane it is a duty increasing in interest with each year's experience to trace out the relationships of present and former patients ... The instances in which two of a family have been under my care are innumerable.*

Even the relatives who come to visit patients frequently display marked forms of neurosis and are in this respect an interesting study to the medico-psychologist.[10]

In November, when the fracture had healed, William Brennan began his exile at Gladesville.

John Brennan was not a particularly strong man: he was open to persuasion by his ill brother and asked for his re-transfer to Callan Park seven months after, in June 1881. William Brennan had made no change in this time, apart from the fact that he now refused to 'occupy himself in any way'. In October of the same year William was discharged to the care of his brother under bond of £20. This money was given to John Brennan to assist in his brother's care and food, and in turn lessened the burden on the state. Again, Manning saw this element of care as integral to what his hospitals could offer:

To subsidize, assist, and encourage the friends of the chronic insane to keep them at home, or to remove them from hospitals when fit for such removal, should, I believe, be part and parcel of our asylum system, and in time I believe a very considerable number will be kept in their homes by means of State, parochial, or municipal aid, but whilst wages are high and there is much scope for active employment, the number will not be large.[11]

In the ensuing four months, the predictable happened: William Brennan's religious delusions, including that 'he was utterly lost forever', returned and he seemed increasingly imbecile. He assaulted his brother and was unable to care for himself. John Brennan took him to Reception House, and William was admitted to Callan Park for the fourth time, more 'demented' than before. He spoke in a 'rambling manner and often [came] to a stop to think and [had] great difficulty expressing himself'.

This yo-yo-ing of Brennan from the care of his brother to Callan Park was an element of Manning's therapy which only those patients with relatives could make use of. In 1886[12] Manning commented 'it has been found possible with safety to allow relatives to remove chronic patients for short periods. No accident has occurred in connection with this system, and the two deaths which occurred during leave were due to natural causes'. After being readmitted in February 1882, Brennan was discharged in April the following year and readmitted in June 1883, after John was obliged to seek police protection due to violence. Brennan's personality began to change: no longer childish and mischievous, he became idle. In 1885 he began writing abusive letters to his brother, saying he was the cause of all of his misfortunes. He told staff that he was suffering from a disease he had caught from the other patients, which was exactly how George Morton felt about him, and had to be restrained at night with muffs to prevent his suicide. Eventually this was upgraded to a camisole, indicating his increasing desperation. In early 1887, William Brennan was again taken out by his brother on bond.

This back and forth admission system was broken eventually by John Brennan's decision to move from Balmain. He became a medical examiner for the AMP Society, travelling the country districts[13] and was later the house surgeon at Hillston Hospital,[14] in the west of New South Wales near the Lachlan River. He was away for many years, only returning in 1904 when he was sixty-seven years old. When he returned he resumed his practice at 338 Darling Street. He lived and worked there for another five years until he died suddenly in 1909. Chronic patient William Brennan, whose hope of discharge died with his brother, lived at Callan Parl until he followed in 1957.

Like Brennan, Jeremiah Lynch[15] was also a patient who was in and out of care during his life. Unlike Brennan though, Lynch had not the kind of family support which would assist him in this. Instead, Lynch was left to his own devices during his more lucid times. Where Brennan was described as a warehouseman or a pawnbroker, both fairly uncomplicated and innocuous jobs, Lynch had been in the New South Wales Artillery. In 1877 the Irish gunner deserted the armed forces and was described in the *Police Gazette*[16] as a tall man with black hair and dark complexion and a forearm tattooed in the form of a wreath and crown, with flowers. He was presumed to have fled to Queensland. Two years later, and while Garryowen House was an uncomplicated asylum with a mere forty-four patients, Lynch was being hunted for the aggravated assault of his wife Margaret.[17] He had been working as a labourer in New South Wales for some time. A warrant for his arrest was issued by the Central Police Branch and he was quickly discovered. He was found guilty and incarcerated in Bathurst Gaol at the beginning of May 1879, where Ah Fuun and Samuel Payne had previously been. While being held at Darlinghurst Gaol questions over his sanity had been clearly raised: Lynch was ordered to undergo an 'exam' in March in the Observation Ward at Darlinghurst Gaol. In September he was released from Bathurst, no further action having been taken as to his sanity, at the end of his four-month sentence. But in November he was arrested again, this time by the Water Police in Sydney, and taken to Reception House.

Presented at Callan Park, he was in a bad way. He was noisy, excited and incoherent of speech. He was dirty in habits like Baroot and Parcelli and 'inclined to be violent'. His constant talking and shouting indicated a severe mania. In terms of bodily health, he was pale and thin and would 'not take his food well'. In Ward Two he was 'noisy and destructive' and secluded for many hours at a time. Like Parcelli and Baroot, his head was blistered in December 1879 but to stop him interfering with his scalp he was forced to wear muffs. His destructive tendencies continued and he was blistered again soon after.

In June 1880 Lynch turned a corner: he was working well with the tailor at Garryowen and was 'apparently quite well'. He was discharged soon after, with the Callan Park staff keen to test his ability to be back in the world. Lynch did well at first. He moved to Forbes and continued working as a tailor for some time until 1886 when he was declared insolvent.[18] Unable to manage his affairs properly, and very poor, Lynch was admitted several times to the Liverpool Asylum in 1895 with chronic bronchitis, and once under the order of the Police Magistrate. The Liverpool Asylum was a government institution which cared for infirm and destitute men; previous to 1862 it had been a branch of the Sydney Benevolent Society. Without any family support Lynch was admitted again to Callan Park in 1905. He stayed less than a year and has left no trace after that.

Both Manning and Blaxland encouraged the old and sickly to be cared for outside the bounds of the hospitals for the insane. Manning's emphasis was always on cure and not merely palliative care: he wanted patients he could help and were *worth* helping because they had lives, family, jobs to return to. In 1887 Manning complained about the patients being fed to his hospitals who could be better treated in poorhouses than in his 'special institutions'. In the same year Blaxland resented nineteen patients added to the swelling wards at his hospital. These were transferred from the Coast Hospital at Little Bay, which had recently changed from a convalescent hospital to a 'fever hospital', treating diseases such as smallpox and tuberculosis. All the men transferred 'were suffering from bodily ailments, and, though undoubtedly mentally deficient, many were cases scarcely requiring treatment in a hospital for the insane'.[19] Lynch's brief return to Callan Park after his time at Liverpool was such a case where unnecessary pressure was put on New South Wales' asylums, as was James Webster's.

James Daniel Webster,[20] also a chronic patient, was a school master in Grafton when he was brought to Reception House in November 1879. Unnecessarily taken to Gladesville to begin with, and then quickly moved to Callan Park, he could not remember his name or address, he did not understand questions he was asked and repeatedly replied 'yes' to everything. He was tremulous and laughed 'unmeaningly'. He was diagnosed with dementia and was described as being 'happy but [his] mind [is] completely gone'. There was nothing which could undo the damage to Webster's brain: only to make him comfortable. This was not what Callan Park was for. Unlike many such men who had no need of the 'specialist' treatment given at Manning's hospitals, Webster was paying £1 12s 6d per month for his treatment. But he was old and hopelessly chronic – and so sense prevailed when he was transferred to one of the Benevolent Asylums in 1886.

In the 1890s Callan Park, originally designed to alleviate the overcrowding of Gladesville and Parramatta, was bursting at the seams with chronic patients. In his *Annual Report* for 1890 Manning wrote that 'The number of patients at the close of the year was 20 in excess of the accommodation ... it is apparent that there must now be a considerable clearing out of the more chronic cases which have accumulated during the twelve years the hospital has been in existence'.[21] In 1891 he recorded that some patients were being forced to sleep in the corridors.[22] In 1892 there was debate in the New South Wales parliament about the 'front of the [Kirkbride] building' which was said to be capable of accommodating 200 patients but was instead being 'monopolised' by the 'half a dozen' medical officers.[23] As a result of this squeeze, many chronic patients were moved to Rydalmere, and some to Parramatta. From 1895 Kenmore also housed such patients.

Many of the original Garryowen patients stayed however – Frederick Legard, who was paying to live in one of the cottages, along with William Brennan and George Merry, were not transferred out but allowed to live out their lives without such a disruption. Such was American Samuel Bennett's[24] happy outcome. Bennett sailed from the USA in 1858 with his wife, onboard the *Castilian,* and they travelled to Grafton together. After some disruption in their marital bliss, Mrs Bennett left her husband and triggered the start of a virulent melancholia in her ex-husband, fired by excessive drinking. He was arrested and taken directly from Darlinghurst Gaol to Gladesville the following year. His illness was put down to 'disappointment in love' and, importantly, intemperance, which had lasted for twenty years. At Gladesville he described himself as single. He worked in the gardens, was silent and reserved and at other times violent. He told staff that he heard voices telling him 'to come away'. Bennett was in the first group of twelve to arrive at Garryowen in 1879 and when he arrived he threw himself into his work. He was a good helper, assisting in the kitchen. Callan Park was his home until he died in 1895 of senile decay.

Bennett and Legard were unusual in their continued residence in Balmain: patients like Lynch who could be discharged, were, and those who could, at least on a trial basis, like Brennan, were, to make room. The medical staff were not nostalgic however: if it was decided that patients could cope with the change, they were removed to another hospital.

Henry Robert Black[25] was a patient in care at Gladesville for twenty years before Manning arrived and so enthralled Henry Parkes. When Black had been first committed to asylum care, manacles and chains had been in vogue to treat the mentally ill in New South Wales. Back then Gladesville's asylum was situated on what was known as 'Bedlam Bay'. There was no Moral Therapy with farms to work or amusements to attend, no classification system: all the patients were thrown in together and left to survive. Records from this time in New South Wales' mental health care are lost now, and questions about their accuracy and detail never to be answered. Black's initial two decades of care, which he shared with Alexander Green, New South Wales' Public Executioner who eventually went mad, are therefore non-existent. The lack of record keeping in the 1850s was highlighted in the 1870s when Black was moved to Garryowen as one of the first forty-four: the staff had no notes as to his initial history, by which they might make a contrast with his current demeanour, to test the progress he had made. They attempted to ask him but 'he himself being much too insane ... [he could not] furnish any' details. He was incoherent, delusional, and gave absurd replies when questioned.

But what the enlightened staff at Callan Park quickly realised was this fifty-two-year-old's genius. He was observed for some time at the early hospital in Ward One. The staff acknowledged the delusions and 'extravagant fancies' which meant he could not be released into the world and which labelled him a chronic maniac, but also saw his strengths:

> *His imagination is of the most inventive kind. He believes that he can make horses out of a piece of skin* [?], *gun-barrel out of rainbows and change men into women at pleasure. He is exceedingly absurd in conversation but is always cheery and good tempered and ready to work, and is at times very useful owing to considerable mechanical genius.*

Black was also frustratingly inconsistent: disoriented in his new surroundings and allowed to work in the park without supervision in 1879, he wandered away and was found in Pyrmont. The medical staff were unimpressed: 'That man who has walked about the grounds for the last three years, wandered away today'. He was found and returned in under two hours. Generally, however, Black was 'allowed much liberty which he [did] not abuse', working in the wards, the grounds and with the Carpenter. In 1888 he escaped briefly, but came back 'voluntarily having ... slept on the ground and got hungry he thought he might come back'. But those who Callan Park had welcomed into its wards in the 1870s and 1880s were not who it could afford to keep in the 1890s. Blaxland needed space for the ever-increasing acutely insane, as Callan Park's role changed in the makeup of the lunatic landscape of New South Wales. Chronic patients were dispersed throughout the state. Black was transferred to Rydalmere in 1890 after a consultation which called him 'demented ... self-satisfied, boastful and incoherent'.

There was always space for acute patients at Callan Park, particularly those suffering from the 'general paralysis of the insane'. These patients were beyond help: but they needed containing while they waited to die of the disease. Unlike the merely demented elderly patients that Manning and Blaxland spurned, these patients were who Callan Park was made, in part, to manage.

John Burton Cox[26] was one such unfortunate man. Described as a 'powerfully built man of fair complexion', Cox was a bricklayer. In 1880, in a demonstration of his increasing violence and paranoia, major characteristics of tertiary syphilis, he was arrested by the police and charged with threatening behaviour. For two years after this he was quiet and contained at home, until in May 1882 the thirty-three-year-old was brought from his home in Newtown to Reception House by his long-suffering wife. Unable to care for her husband while bringing up five children, Mrs Cox could only turn to Manning's hospital system for help. At the Reception House at Darlinghurst he was violent and troublesome and attempted escape. At Callan Park it was noted that he was experiencing difficulty in speaking, which he would engage in at random. With delusions of grandeur, he would boast of the contracts he was working on and the number of men he employed, and then burst into tears. He said, 'that he wished to collect all the bones in the neighbourhood to crush and make a disinfectant by means of a brick machine; that he had numbers of policemen and prisoners working for him, that he wanted to be cupped and that he had large sums of money paid to him'. Staff at Callan Park recognised him as a previous patient of Gladesville Hospital. Cox would not be released again.

He was violent and destructive: three days into his care he was confined to a camisole to stop him from destroying his clothing and the windows. He was involved in fights with other patients and received a black eye during one. In July 1882 Mrs Cox made a complaint, which demonstrated her inability to accept the realities of her husband's disease:

> *Mrs Cox, wife of L* [sic] *Burton Cox a patient here, complained today that her husband has been ill-treated by the attendants and mentioned in proof that his left arm above the elbow was bruised and had a large tender swelling on the inside. On investigation I found evident exaggeration to say nothing of the gross mendacity of the complaint. There was no bruising or evidence of it, the swelling was a small abscess of the lymphatic gland which ... evidently resulted from a small abrasion ...*

Cox's treatment was expensive, with an attendant allocated to watch him day and night, for his own and others' safety. Three months before his death in December 1882, Cox was deeply unwell, but clearly in the right institution for his condition:

> *Black eye reported at rounds ... attendant Carter was minding* [Cox] *as he sat in an easy chair when he struggled very much to get up and attack another patient and struck his eye against the chair. Patient is a general paralytic and an attendant has to ... look after him when he is up, in consequence of his extreme restlessness and mischievous propensity. I have no reason to suppose he was struck by Carter against whom I have never heard a complaint. The patient is too demented to say how it occurred.*

The impact of mental illness on the families of sufferers in this time was not well documented, though imagination might give us insight into Mrs Cox's reaction to her young husband's decline. The heart break with which John Brennan re-admitted his brother over the years was not recorded either and we are left to imagine what frustration and sadness he must have felt. Not everyone was as cold hearted as Frederick Legard's nephew. What did Fillipo Parcelli's pregnant wife feel when her husband was taken in a straightjacket to Gladesville for the first time? Most saddened must have been the wife of Thomas Manning,[27] a printer and publisher based in Dubbo. Suffering from dementia caused by intemperance and epilepsy, when he was brought to Callan Park he could not always recognise her. Staff were mystified by his illness:

> *His condition is a peculiar one. He reads to himself and to fellow patients for hours together, with proper instruction and apparently with full understanding of the subject, but does not remember the smallest item ten minutes afterwards. In the same way his whole past existence is a blank, and when visited by his wife he appears glad to see her, talks to her and yet within a few minutes is unconscious that she has ever been near him.*

Any relief Mrs Cox found from the final decease of her husband was not for long however: syphilis being hereditary, her son, Thomas B. Cox, was also a sufferer, as discussed in the New South Wales parliament some years later:

> *I wish to draw the attention of the Minister to the case of Thomas B. Cox, a prisoner in Berrima Gaol. This man was originally a Vernon boy, and has served thirty-eight months in the gaol, twenty-six of which were spent in solitary confinement in the cells. He has also served twenty-seven days in the blackhole on bread and water, and has been flogged three times. The result of the punishment, however, has only been to make him worse. I may mention that the prisoner's father died in the lunatic asylum at Callan Park, and that those who have to deal with him think he is more a subject for a lunatic asylum than for a prison. I wish to know if, under the circumstances, the Minister will cause an examination to be made by medical experts to find out if this man is insane or not.*[28]

Callan Park could not help everyone. Violent aggressors like Cox are difficult to sympathise with, particularly with Mrs Cox making the staff's lives difficult through her meddling and accusations. Patients like John Evans evoke our sympathy easily however: kind and gentle, and struggling to belong in the strange new place that was Australia.

John Evans[29] was born in 1841 in England. By the time he was thirty-nine he was suffering from severe melancholia. A tall man, 'thin and delicate looking', with dark hair and whiskers and a forlorn expression, Evans sought help at Gladesville Asylum. He suffered from some lung disease which gave him a persistent cough, along with a minor level of deafness. He was severely depressed, and under the impression that 'he ha[d] enemies in Sydney who are plotting against him and [would] not allow him to live here, that he [was] persecuted by them'. Never inclined to violence, Evans was always clean and quiet. Resident at Gladesville for six months, he was discharged in the hope that he could restart his career as a sail maker. Evans' plan was to take a ship to the warmer climate of Fiji to restore his bodily health. But unable to find passage there and in decreasing health and spirits, he surrendered himself to the police in the form of constable Charles Hedges who took him to Reception House.

Shy and retiring, Evans was brought in March 1880 to Callan Park. He was an ideal patient: housed in Ward Two but without the need for restraint, Evans had a good prognosis. He worked daily in the store with Legard and Merry, and 'never referre[d] to his delusions'. He was on the way to recovery, and the staff of Callan Park would have been optimistic about this. But the work Evans was praised for by the staff was to be his undoing: in May that year he took a knife from the store. 'He left ... taking with him a knife with which he attempted to open a vein in his left arm. This failed and he then threw himself into the water near the garden fence[. H]e was at once rescued by the gardener [Cheetham] and brought home. He was cold and weak'. Hot brandy was given to him and staff were hopeful of a recovery; but his breathing became laboured and on the evening of 20 May this gentle soul died of pneumonia.

EPILOGUE

I first visited Callan Park in July 2015 when I attended a course there at the New South Wales Writers' Centre. Like many Sydney-siders I had never heard of Callan Park before and had no idea of its history. Walking down the drive and making my way to a little concrete seat on the edge of what I now know as Garryowen House, I was struck by the atmosphere which permeates the park. There is something so still and calm in those grounds. A sensitivity exists there which was not impacted by the dozens of people who walked past me, tugging their dogs along with them. There is a presence in the site – not ghosts or spirits of patients, nothing so macabre – and you can see just by visiting what Manning and Parkes also saw in it.

It wasn't until my fourth or fifth class at the Writers' Centre that I googled the place. I remembered vaguely my Year Six teacher – not the most stable of individuals – repeatedly threatening my class with a permanent trip 'to Rozelle' whenever we did something which annoyed him. I read about the site on Wikipedia and then found the Friends of Callan Park's website. I had already read a great deal about Victorian-era asylums in England, sparked initially by my love of *Jane Eyre*. I took myself off that afternoon for a walk around the circumference of Kirkbride. I came to it from the back and was very excited to identify the ha-ha walls which I had read about in other books.

I gathered up the courage one day to go into the Kirkbride Complex itself. I saw the shaded verandahs, the large green spaces, the stained-glass chapel window. I wondered what kinds of people had been there and what it had been like in those early days. My disappointment that no history of Callan Park had already been written was eclipsed by my excitement that I could make such a project *my* job. And so I found out about the first men of Callan Park, leaning for a year over the dusty volumes which were once to be found in Blaxland's office and are now in the State Records Authority in Kingswood, New South Wales.

When I began my research I had very firmly in my head the terrible Bertha Mason from *Jane Eyre*, the unbalanced and isolated John Perceval, and a whole host of other knowledge about Victorian asylums and psychiatric care – all fairly grim – propped up with scenes from films like *Girl, Interrupted*. My many misconceptions about Victorian asylums I shared with those irate neighbours of Callan Park from 1876, and when I started researching I admit that that was what I was hoping for: brutal treatment, fear, humiliation. But in researching Manning and the jewel in his crown – Callan Park – I found a truly humane and benevolent doctor and institution. Yes, there was the occasional brutal or ill-considering attendant walking the corridors, throwing his weight around – but there were also dozens of staff who were caring and devoted to the men and women in their charge.

I am like John Keep, that irate neighbour, who came to be seduced by the standard of care offered by his neighbourhood asylum. In 1879, only recently a petitioner and fearful father and husband, he presented to the patients of Callan Park an emu to add to the growing menagerie housed at the asylum for the rehabilitation of patients. Two years after that, completely enamoured with the place, he was providing baskets of fruit from his own orchards.[1] This book, full of biographies of men of no particular achievement, but who are interesting for that very reason, is my donation to the first patients of early Callan Park.

There is something quite magical about visiting Callan Park now that I know what I know, and I hope you feel the same. When you see the gardens, you know that William Andrews and Paul Littel planted them first. When you look at the bay at the bottom of the hill, do you not see Parcelli running for freedom? When you see the sandstone gardener's cottage on the grassy slope, do not you think of Cheetham and his son, the first outdoor attendant? When you look at the verandah linking Garryowen to the little cottage beside it, cannot you see Frederick Legard sitting there, happily working at his arithmetic in the sun?

APPENDICES

1. THE ORIGINAL 'FORTY-FOUR' OFFICIALLY TRANSFERRED TO THE NEW HOSPITAL FOR THE INSANE, CALLAN PARK, 1 AUGUST 1878

John Fowler, a 49-year-old single porter from Ireland, lately living in Sydney. He suffered from dementia caused by drink and in 1893 was transferred to Rydalmere as a chronic patient.

Henry Robert Black, a Protestant 52-year-old single shoemaker from New South Wales, lately living in Bathurst. He suffered from delusional mania and in 1894 was transferred to Rydalmere as a chronic patient.

George Bates, a Protestant 61-year-old labourer from England, lately living in Sydney. He suffered from melancholia and his sister was also insane. He died in 1881 at Callan Park.

Charles Regan, a Catholic 53-year-old dealer from Ireland, lately living in Sydney. Married, he suffered from mania as a result of a diseased brain. His mother and father were also insane. He died in 1889 from senile decay at Callan Park.

Patrick Kearney, a Catholic 40-year-old from New South Wales, lately living in Sydney. He suffered from imbecility, caused by epilepsy and was insane from birth. His mother was also insane. In 1893 he was transferred to Rydalmere.

Thomas Smythe, a Protestant 51-year-old labourer from England, lately in living in Sydney. He suffered from delusional mania and died in 1891 at Callan Park from a carcinoma of the stomach.

William Goodwin, a Catholic 57-year-old labourer from Ireland, lately living in Sydney. He suffered from delusional mania and in 1887 became feeble and died.

John Sullivan, a Catholic 43-year-old labourer from Ireland, lately living in Windsor. He suffered from mania and died in 1889 from dementia and progressive muscular dystrophy.

John Barragay (alias Ryan, alias Scully), a Catholic 46-year-old labourer from Ireland, lately living in Penrith. He suffered from chronic mania and died in 1894.

William Aitkenhead, a Catholic 39-year-old wheelwright from New South Wales, lately living in Sydney. He was married with two children and suffered from chronic mania after an injury to his head. He died in 1895 from exhaustion caused by diarrhoea at Callan Park.

Alfred Cooper, a Protestant 55-year-old tutor from England, lately living in Sydney. He was married and suffered from delusional mania.

Joseph Edwards, a Protestant 27-year-old from England, lately living in Sydney. He suffered from hereditary imbecility and epilepsy. He died in 1890 at Callan Park.

Henry Hamill, a Catholic 39-year-old labourer from Ireland, lately living in Sydney. He suffered from chronic mania and was transferred back to Gladesville in 1884.

Josias Keenan, a Protestant 46-year-old from Ireland, lately living in Sydney. He was married and suffered from dementia after a fall from a verandah. He died at Callan Park in 1890.

Joseph R Brown, a Protestant 67-year-old storekeeper from England, lately living in Musselbrook. He suffered from melancholia and received extra rations of rum and beer for the work he carried out at Callan Park.

William Holley, a Protestant 57-year-old coal miner from Wales, lately living in Newcastle. He suffered from mania and in 1895 was transferred to Kenmore.

George Alexander Macfie, a Protestant 35-year-old from New South Wales, lately living in Petersham. He suffered from hereditary imbecility and epilepsy. He died in 1886 at Callan Park.

John Fahey (alias Foley, alias Mickey Roche), a Catholic 33-year-old labourer from Ireland, lately living in Tamworth. He suffered from general insanity first observed in Tamworth Gaol. In 1895 he was transferred to Kenmore.

Alfred Chandler, a Catholic 31-year-old labourer from New South Wales, lately living in Grafton. He suffered from dementia caused by the death of his father due to cancer.

Peter Baxter, a Protestant 35-year-old labourer from New South Wales, lately living in Campbelltown. He suffered from delusional mania and died in 1903 at Callan Park.

Matthew Spencer, a Protestant 72-year-old shepherd from England, lately having been resident at the Benevolent Asylum at Parramatta. He had only one arm, and also suffered from dementia. In 1885 was transferred back to the Benevolent Asylum.

Robert Boon, a Protestant 28-year-old carrier from England, living lately in Mirramundi. He suffered from dementia caused by a stroke and in 1879 was transferred back to Gladesville.

Frederick Legard, a Protestant 65-year-old clergyman from England, lately living in Sydney. He suffered from chronic mania and died in 1897 from senile decay at Callan Park.

John Egan, a Catholic 27-year-old farmer from Ireland, lately living in Ulladulla. He suffered from dementia and his sister was admitted to Gladesville in 1887.

John Randall, a Protestant 60-year-old jobber from England, lately living in Camperdown. He suffered from mania due to a combination of epilepsy and a head injury. In 1885 he died at Callan Park following a bout of severe diarrhoea.

Henry Smith, a Protestant 65-year-old dealer from England, lately living in Mudgee. He suffered from delusional mania and in 1885 was transferred to the Benevolent Asylum.

Michael Lahey, a Catholic 40-year-old farmer from New South Wales, lately living in Mudgee. Labelled as having been an imbecile from birth, he was transferred to Parramatta.

Ah Chun, a Pagan 26-year-old sailor from China, lately living in Sydney. He suffered from dementia and was discharged in 1882.

Edward Cusak, a Catholic 64-year-old farmer from Ireland, lately living in Morpeth. He was a widower suffering from melancholia. In 1880 he was discharged as cured under the care of his son.

Thomas Mannering, a Catholic 38-year-old printer and publisher from New South Wales, lately living in Dubbo. He had four children and suffered from dementia and epilepsy. He died in 1879 at Callan Park.

Thomas Feehan, a Catholic 27-year-old labourer from New South Wales, lately living in Braidwood. Suffering from imbecility from birth, he died at Callan Park in 1890.

John Budge, a Protestant 33-year-old tailor from Scotland, lately living in Sydney. He suffered from delusional mania and, a widower, had three children.

Dennis Thomas, a Catholic 44-year-old farmer from New South Wales, lately living in Newcastle. He suffered from delusional mania caused by a horse which fell on him as a 22 year old. He was discharged on bond from Callan Park in 1879.

Daniel Robinson, a Catholic 50-year-old publican from Ireland, lately living in Sydney. He was married with twelve children and suffered from dementia brought about by intemperance. He died in 1884 after a severe bout of diarrhoea at Callan Park.

David Attaway, a Protestant 67-year-old farmer from England, lately living in Orange. He was a widower and suffered from delusional melancholia. He died at Callan Park in 1880 from a combination of senile decay and bladder disease.

Thomas Crotty, a Catholic 57-year-old labourer from Ireland, lately living in Sydney. He was a widower and suffered from dementia due to ill health. He had five children and an insane cousin, and died in 1880 at Callan Park.

James Jamieson, a Protestant 44-year-old carpenter from Scotland, lately living in Redfern. He suffered from melancholia. He had five children and was eventually discharged under a bond of £3 to the care of his wife.

Simon Patrick Holland, a Catholic 39-year-old from Ireland. He was married with five children and was a publican. Suffering from delusional melancholia, he was transferred to Parramatta in 1891.

Patrick Keely, a Catholic 60-year-old farmer from Ireland, lately living in Moruya. He suffered from mania due to epilepsy and was married with five children. He died suddenly in 1880 at Callan Park.

George Merry, a Protestant 50-year-old miner from England, lately living in Sydney. He suffered from melancholia brought about by ill health. Discharged as recovered in 1880, he was soon readmitted and died at Callan Park in 1895.

Henry Jones, a Protestant 61-year-old bank clerk from England, lately living in Sydney. He suffered from dementia due to intemperance and died in 1903.

Henry Vickery, a Protestant 68-year-old labourer from England, lately living in Queenbeyan. He suffered from dementia and was transferred to the Asylum for the Destitute at Liverpool in 1881.

James Leebeter, a Protestant 48-year-old farmer from New South Wales, lately living in Carcoar. He suffered from delusional melancholia thought to be hereditary since his father was also insane. He was married with six children and was discharged in 1884.

Charles Cook, a Protestant 59-year-old labourer from England, lately living in Bundarrn. He suffered from dementia and epilepsy and was discharged from Callan Park in 1881.

2. MEN TRANSFERRED FROM GLADESVILLE TO THE NEW HOSPITAL FOR THE INSANE, CALLAN PARK, 12 SEPTEMBER 1879

Samuel Bennett, a Protestant 46-year-old sawyer from the United States, lately living in Grafton. He suffered from melancholia due to a disappointment in love, and intemperance. He died in 1895 of senile decay at Callan Park.

Henry Glannon, a Protestant 27-year-old butcher from New South Wales, lately living in Balmain. He suffered from mania due to epilepsy and died at Callan Park in 1887.

Joseph Allen, a Baptist 22-year-old gardener from New South Wales, lately living in Waterloo. He suffered from mania caused by pubescence. In 1889 he was transferred to Newcastle.

John Cane, a Catholic 33-year-old engineer from Ireland, lately living in Mudgee. He suffered from dementia due to brain disease and was discharged as cured in 1880.

Martin Ryan, a Catholic 25-year-old labourer from New South Wales, lately living in Queenbeyan. He was melancholic and worked well at Callan Park, receiving additional allowances of beef tea and rum. He died at Callan Park in 1881.

John Dye, a Protestant 51-year-old carpenter from England, lately living at the Benevolent Asylum in Liverpool. He suffered from dementia caused by brain disease. He died at Callan Park in 1883 from senile decay and exhaustion.

Lewis O'Leary, a Catholic 21-year-old medical student from Ireland, lately living in Singleton. He suffered from delusional melancholia and in 1893 was transferred as a chronic patient to Rydalmere.

Thomas Ryan, a Catholic 35-year-old mason from Ireland, lately living in Sydney. He suffered from melancholia supposedly caused by syphilis. He was married with three children and in 1891 was transferred to Parramatta.

Joseph C Orton, a Catholic 41-year-old labourer from England, lately living in Bathurst. He suffered from delusional mania due to isolation. He was discharged from Callan Park in 1885.

G I Hamblin, a Protestant 35-year-old sawyer from England, lately living in Sydney. He suffered from dementia due to epilepsy. He died at Callan Park in 1888 as the result of a seizure.

Joseph Clegg, a Protestant 39-year-old draper from Lancashire in England, lately living in Burwood. He was married with eleven children and suffered from mania.

Thomas Clark, a Protestant 44-year-old from King's Country, Ireland, lately living in Brookong in Wagga Wagga. He was married and suffered from delusional mania. He died at Callan Park in 1897.

3. MEN TRANSFERRED FROM GLADESVILLE TO THE NEW HOSPITAL FOR THE INSANE, CALLAN PARK, 26 SEPTEMBER 1879

Justice Sipple, a Protestant 35-year-old fencer from Germany, lately living in Bogan River. He suffered from melancholia and was discharged from Callan Park in 1888 after he escaped.

George Forster, a Protestant 39-year-old farmer from New South Wales, lately living in Maitland. He suffered from dementia and had an insane uncle. He was discharged from Callan Park in 1890.

Eli Knowles, a Protestant 28-year-old seaman from England, lately living in Bathurst. He suffered from a hereditary form of dementia, his cousin also being insane. In 1891 he was transferred to Parramatta.

John Baly, a Protestant 25-year-old labourer from New South Wales, lately living in Maitland. He suffered from delusional melancholia. In 1895 he was transferred as a chronic patient to Rydalmere.

Charles E Johnston, a Protestant 29-year-old farmer from England, lately living in Casino. He suffered from sub-acute mania and in 1892 was transferred to Rydalmere.

James R Clayton, a Protestant 24-year-old blacksmith from New South Wales, lately living in Balmain. He suffered from delusional melancholia due to sunstroke.

John Adams, a Protestant 30-year-old miner from England, lately living in Scone. He suffered from delusional melancholia. He died at Callan Park in 1885.

James Martin, a Protestant 24-year-old sailor from Ireland, lately living in Tamworth. He suffered from delusional melancholia.

Samuel Wade, a Methodist 39-year-old farmer from England, lately living in Sydney. He suffered from dementia caused by epilepsy. In 1893 he was transferred as a chronic patient to Rydalmere.

Patrick Gillam, a Catholic 41-year-old labourer from Ireland, lately living in Orange. He was married and suffered from melancholia. In 1884 he was transferred to Parramatta.

Terence McGuire, a Catholic 36-year-old cassier from Ireland, lately living in Orange. He suffered from delusional melancholia. In 1891 he was transferred to Parramatta.

William Sleumaker, a Catholic 30-year-old shoemaker from New South Wales, lately living in Sydney. He suffered from delusional melancholia caused by intemperance and hereditary taint, as his mother was also insane. In 1894 he was transferred to Rydalmere.

4. MEN TRANSFERRED FROM GLADESVILLE TO THE NEW HOSPITAL FOR THE INSANE, CALLAN PARK, 6 OCTOBER 1879

Dennis O'Connor, a Catholic 39-year-old farmer from New South Wales, lately living in Hamley. He suffered from dementia after he fell from a horse. He died at Callan Park in 1889 from exhaustion.

Henry Jollis, a Protestant 27-year-old boot finisher from New South Wales, lately living in Waterloo. He suffered from mania caused by epilepsy. In 1893 he was transferred as a chronic patient to Rydalmere.

Terence MacCusker, a Catholic 39-year-old labourer from Ireland, lately living in Bathurst. He suffered from dementia.

James Dunne, a Catholic 23-year-old machine ruler from New South Wales, lately living in Sydney. He suffered from mania brought about by epilepsy. He died at Callan Park in 1886.

Amos Pearse, a Protestant 57-year-old tailor from England. He suffered from mania caused by epilepsy. He was married with nine children and in 1893 was transferred to Rydalmere.

Unknown Man (alias Thomas McMahon), a 29-year-old from New South Wales, lately living in Armidale. He suffered from melancholia. He died in 1881 at Callan Park.

William Jones, a Protestant 42-year-old sawyer from England, lately living in Mudgee. He was married with five children and suffered from dementia. In 1881 he died at Callan Park.

William Andrews, a Protestant 29-year-old labourer from New South Wales, lately living in Orange. He suffered from mania caused by epilepsy. He was transferred as a chronic patient to Rydalmere in 1893.

William Clancy, a Catholic 35-year-old butcher from New South Wales, lately living in Cook's River. He suffered from dementia caused by intemperance. He was married with five children. In 1896 he died at Callan Park from a cerebral haemorrhage.

Fillipo Parcelli (alias Parcellie, Tomassini, Phillipo Parcelli), a Protestant 26-year-old labourer from Italy, lately living in Young. He suffered from mania and was transferred back to Gladesville in 1882.

George Wilson, a Catholic 49-year-old labourer from Ireland, lately living in Tamworth. He suffered from delusional melancholia. He died at Callan Park in 1889.

Alexander Clubb, a Protestant 31-year-old plasterer from Scotland, lately living in Pyrmont. He suffered from mania and died in 1919 at Callan Park.

5. MEN TRANSFERRED FROM GLADESVILLE TO THE NEW HOSPITAL FOR THE INSANE, CALLAN PARK, 10 DECEMBER 1879

Samuel Payne, a Protestant 51-year-old labourer from England, lately living in Forbes. He suffered from delusional melancholia due to a lonely life. In 1898 he was transferred to Kenmore.

Michael Scanlinn, a Catholic 39-year-old bus driver from Ireland, lately living in Waverley. He suffered from delusional melancholia. He worked well at Callan Park, receiving additional allowances of brandy and beer. He was married with four children and was discharged in 1880.

Joshua Fitzpatrick, a Catholic 22-year-old saddler from Victoria, lately living in Sydney. He suffered from hereditary delusional melancholia. In 1880 he was transferred to Parramatta.

Thomas Robson, a Protestant 24-year-old seaman from England, lately living in Sydney. He suffered from dementia caused by epilepsy. He died at Callan Park in 1884.

William Williams (alias Crook), a Protestant 32-year-old labourer from England, lately living in Nundle. He suffered from delusional mania. In 1894 he was transferred as a chronic patient to Rydalmere.

George A G Brinchley, a Protestant 43-year-old labourer from England. Married, he suffered from the 'general paralysis of the insane', and his father, brother and sister were also insane. He died at Callan Park in 1880.

Daniel Henry, a Catholic 46-year-old from Scotland, lately living in Armidale. Married with seven children, he suffered from the 'general paralysis of the insane'. In 1881 he died at Callan Park.

James Clarke, a Protestant 43-year-old labourer from England, lately living in Newcastle. He was married with three children. He suffered from mania and in 1890 was transferred as a chronic patient to Parramatta.

Paul Guichery, a Catholic 35-year-old seaman from France, lately living in Newcastle. He suffered from mania.

Chan Long, a Pagan 39-year-old miner from China, lately living in Sydney. He suffered from acute mania. He died at Callan Park in 1884.

Charles Stacey, a Protestant 46-year-old builder from England, lately living in Sydney. He was married with four children and suffered from dementia caused by epilepsy. He died at Callan Park in 1880.

James Daniel Webster, a Protestant school master lately living in Grafton. He suffered from dementia and in 1886 was transferred to the Benevolent Asylum.

NOTES

Preface

1 'Proposed Lunatic Asylum at Garryowen: Petition Against – Landowners and Others', *NSW Legislative Assembly Votes and Proceedings*, Session 1875/76 – Vol. 6, p. 101, 8 March 1876.

2 Ibid., p. 103, 31 March 1876.

3 The signatures of both petitions have sadly been lost. However, several other petitions and their signatures survive. See State Records Authority of New South Wales: *NRS 906, Colonial Secretary Special Bundles: Erection of Callan Park Lunatic Asylum, 1873–79* [4/818.3].

4 See 'Parliamentary Debates', *Victorian Hansard,* 11 January 1859, and 'Tenth Report of the Printing Committee', *Victorian Legislative Assembly*, 20 January 1859.

5 'More Callan Park Allegations: Order for Royal Commission', *Canberra Times,* 8 December 1960.

6 'Royal Commission Refused: Inquiry into Callan Park', *Newcastle Sun,* 19 July 1948.

7 'Callan Park: Indictment by Judge in Report', *Canberra Times,* 8 September 1961.

8 For example, Mitchell Toy, 'Victorian psychiatric patients' grim fate in hellish 1800s hospitals', *Herald Sun,* 9 December 2014, and Ben Pike 'Sydney's shameful asylums: The silent houses of pain where inmates were chained and sadists reigned', *Daily Telegraph,* 2 March 2015.

Note on the Sources

1 Stephen Garton, *Medicine and Madness. A Social History of Insanity in NSW 1880–1940*, (Kensington: New South Wales University Press, 1988), pp. 101–2.

1. Callan Park: Branch Establishment and the 'First Forty-Four'

1 Sources for Frederick Legard, unless otherwise cited, are: SRANSW, NRS 5019, *Reception House Medical Case Book* [11/2152]; NRS 5031, *Gladesville Medical Case Book* [4/8153], NRS 5047, *Gladesville Addresses of Patients' Friends* [4/10565]; NRS 4994, *Callan Park Medical Case Book* [3/4652]; NRS 4998, *Callan Park Medical Journal* [3/7045]; NRS 4984, *Callan Park Case Papers 1878–1882* [3/3317]; NRS 12252 and 12253, *Master in Lunacy Maintenance Ledgers* and *Books* [3/14224–7; 3/14229].

2 *Sydney Morning Herald,* 1 September 1877.

3 'Callan Park', *Evening News,* 7 July 1876.

4 Ibid.

5 SRANSW, NRS 4984, *Callan Park Case Papers 1878–1882* [3/3317].

6 Pasquin, 'The Social Kaleidoscope: No. 17 The Callan Park Lunatic Asylum, Section II', *Freeman's Journal,* 10 July 1880.

7 Historic Houses Trust, *Caroline Simpson Library & Research Collection* [L2006/8].

8 Manning, *1881 Annual Report of the Inspector General of the Insane* (Sydney: Government Printer, 1882).

9 Manning, *1882 Annual Report of the Inspector General of the Insane* (Sydney: Government Printer, 1883).

10 Pasquin, 'The Social Kaleidoscope'.

11 Ibid.

12 'Callan Park'.

13 Pasquin, 'The Social Kaleidoscope'.

14 Manning, *1882 Annual Report of the Inspector General of the Insane.*

15 Pasquin, 'The Social Kaleidoscope'. At some point the Edith Wright Room was also painted in this manner. Such a pattern has been recently revealed on one wall of this room and can be viewed under glass there.

16 'Callan Park. A Great State Institution', *Sydney Mail,* 12 August 1903; photographs by Alfred Small, [Photographs of Callan Park Mental Hospital, 1903], Call Number [PX*D 241], State Library New South Wales.

17 Manning, *1881 Annual Report of the Inspector General of the Insane.*

18 Ibid.

19 Manning, *1882 Annual Report of the Inspector General of the Insane.*

20 For example, Manning, *1882 Annual Report of the Inspector General of the Insane.*

21 Pasquin, 'The Social Kaleidoscope'.

22 Manning, *1881 Annual Report of the Inspector General of the Insane.*

23 *Sydney Morning Herald,* 23 November 1881.

24 Deaths of Prominent Queenslanders', *Evening News,* 9 July 1898.

25 Manning, *1882 Annual Report of the Inspector General of the Insane* and *1883 Annual Report of the Inspector General of the Insane* (Sydney: Government Printer, 1884).

26 SRANSW, NRS 5001, *Callan Park Correspondence from Patients,* George Morton [3/4921].

27 SRANSW, NRS 906, *Colonial Secretary Special Bundles: Erection of Callan Park Lunatic Asylum, 1873–79* [4/818.3], *The Colonial Architect to the Under Secretary for Public Works Submitting plans for the temporary accommodation at Callan Park, 13 June 1877.*

28 SRANSW, NRS 5043, *Gladesville Medical Journal* [8/2326B].

29 As described in Ray and Richard Beckett, *Hangman: The Life and Times of Alexander Green Public Executioner to the Colony of New South Wales* (Melbourne: Nelson, 1980).

30 In January 1875 there were a series of letters to the editor of the *Sydney Morning Herald* on this topic, including a response from Manning: *Sydney Morning Herald,* January 1, 5 and 8, 1875.

31 See SRANSW, NRS 4998, *Callan Park Medical Journal* [3/7045] and individual patients' *Medical Case Books*.

32 Manning, *1882 Annual Report of the Inspector General of the Insane* and *1883 Annual Report of the Inspector General of the Insane.*

33 Manning, *Address Delivered on Resigning Charge as Medical Superintendent of the Hospitals for the Insane at Gladesville and Callan Park*, (Sydney: Gibbs, Shallard, & Co., 1879), p. 7.

34 See SRANSW, NRS 4994, *Callan Park Medical Case Book* [3/4652] and NRS 5066, *Newcastle Medical Case Book* [34/3483].

35 I am indebted to Jenny Pearce at The King's School Archive for this information.

36 'The Late Dr. Blaxland', *Sydney Mail*, 27 April 1904.

37 [Family and holiday album, 1899–1908/ Arthur Whitling], Call Number [PXE 917], State Library New South Wales.

38 For example, 'Government Gazette', *Sydney Morning Herald*, 22 January 1887.

39 'Horticultural Society of New South Wales', *Sydney Morning Herald*, 24 October 1889.

40 For example, the *Australian Town and Country Journal*, 12 November 1881, reported that Blaxland made eleven runs, and his team, Gladesville, won.

41 The cricket paddock, which is today a soccer oval, was extended in 1883 (Manning, *1883 Annual Report of the Inspector General of the Insane*) and in 1892 a taller fence was erected for the privacy of sportsmen from the public who were prone to stop and jeer at patients, along with a pavilion which containing dressing rooms and seats for spectators (Manning, *1892 Annual Report of the Inspector General of the Insane* (Sydney: Government Printer, 1893)).

42 Manning, *1882 Annual Report of the Inspector General of the Insane.*

43 Manning, *1883 Annual Report of the Inspector General of the Insane.*

44 Ibid.

45 Manning, *1882 Annual Report of the Inspector General of the Insane.*

46 Manning, *1881 Annual Report of the Inspector General of the Insane.*

47 Manning, *1882 Annual Report of the Inspector General of the Insane.*

48 Manning, *1883 Annual Report of the Inspector General of the Insane.*

2. The Mental State of Australia

1 Report published in the *Sydney Morning Herald*, 24 May 1877.

2 'Hospitals for the Insane', *Weekly Times*, 7 July 1877.

3 Report published in the *Sydney Morning Herald*, 24 May 1877.

4 Frederic Norton Manning, *The Causation and Prevention of Insanity*, (Sydney: Government Printer, 1880), p. 13.

5 Summary of 'Report' published in the *Sydney Morning Herald*, 23 April 1877.

6 James Digby Legard, *The Legards of Anlaby & Ganton: Their Neighbours & Neighbourhood*, (London: Simpkin, Marshall, Hamilton, Kent & Co., 1926), p. 109.

7 East Riding Archives (ERA), 'Insanity of Thomas and William Legard' [DDGR/43/17/12].

8 ERA, 'Thomas Legard placed in madhouse' [DDGR/43/17/24].

9 See *Alumni Carthusiani* (a list of Charterhouse graduates) and the *Charterhouse Register 1769–1872.*

10 The National Archives UK (TNA), [C 211/15/L90] 'Sir Thomas Legard, bart of Ganton, Yorkshire: commission and inquisition of lunacy, into his state of mind and his property'.

11 Legard, *The Legards of Anlaby and Ganton*, p. 116.

12 Ibid., p. 121.

13 A H Tod, *Charterhouse*, (London: George Bell and Sons, 1900), pp. 16–17.

14 Anthony Trollope, (ed John Morley), *Thackeray. English Men of Letters Series,* (London: Macmillan, 1879), pp. 4-5.

15 I am indebted to Catherine Smith, the archivist for Charterhouse School for this information.

16 I am indebted to Amanda Goode, Emmanuel College archivist, for this information.

17 Records of study at Cambridge for Legard's period are largely lost; his *senior optime* result was used in an advertisement for the Victorian Collegiate Institution, where Legard taught in Melbourne (*Argus,* 1 January 1864).

18 Borthwick Institute for Archives, University of York, *Institution Act Book* INST/AB/20, pp. 322, 345, 352 and *Ordination papers* ORD/P/1839 and ORD/D/1840.

19 I am indebted to Helen Clark at the East Riding Archive for this information, which was gathered from the *Registers of Ganton 1846–1852.*

20 TNA, [MH 94/1-47] 'UK Lunacy Patients Admission Registers, 1846–1912', admission no. 8314.

21 TNA, [HO 107] 'Census Returns' (1851).

22 Legard, *The Legards of Anlaby and Ganton,* p. 140.

23 Borthwick Institute for Archives, University of York, *Cecilia Legard of Bramham (Prog),* February 1855.

24 Legard, *The Legards of Anlaby and Ganton,* p. 139.

25 Pasquin, 'The Social Kaleidoscope'.

26 Including Cremorne and Pascoevale [*sic,* Pasco Vale] Asylums; advertisement in the *Sydney Mail,* 10 February 1866.

27 'Unorthodox Sydney. By a Pilgrim. No. 8 Bay View House Lunatic Asylum', *Freeman's Journal,* 7 July 1877.

28 The New Norfolk Insane Asylum in Tasmania, which opened in 1827, was built specifically to contain lunatics in Van Diemen's Land. It was quickly dwarfed by Tarban Creek however, whose influence could be seen throughout New South Wales and Victoria in the nineteenth century, while New Norfolk remained fairly contained and isolated from developments throughout Australia.

29 Frederick Norton Manning, *Report on Lunatic Asylums* (Sydney: Government Printer, 1868), p. 157.

30 *NSW Legislative Assembly* transcript, 26 October 1893.

31 Manning, *Report on Lunatic Asylums*, p. 158.

32 Frederic Norton Manning, *Address in Psychological Medicine* (Sydney: Government Printer, 1888), p. 15; Manning, *Report on Lunatic Asylums*, p. 217.

33 'A Month in Kew Asylum and Yarra Bend', *Argus*, 22 July 1876.

34 'Death of Dr F N Manning', *Sydney Mail and New South Wales Advertiser*, 24 June 1903.

35 Henry Parkes, *Fifty Years in the Making of Australian History*, (North Carolina: Hayes Barton Press, 2006), pp. 167–8.

36 Frederic Norton Manning, *Address Delivered on Resigning Charge as Medical Superintendent of the Hospitals for the Insane at Gladesville and Callan Park*, p. 5.

37 In 1883 patient Keenan's shoulder was dislocated after an altercation with another patient (SRANSW, NRS 4998, *Callan Park Medical Journal* [3/7045]).

38 For example: vaccinations are noted in Manning, *1881 Annual Report of the Inspector General of the Insane*; in 1881 an emergency tracheotomy was performed, without success, on patient John Henry and in 1883 patient H. Bogan was given stitches by Blaxland (both SRANSW, NRS 4998, *Callan Park Medical Journal* [3/7045]); over the summer of 1885/6 parts of the hospital were used to treat an outbreak of typhoid fever in the staff (Manning, *1885 Annual Report of the Inspector General of the Insane* (Sydney: Government Printer, 1886)).

39 Manning, *Report on Lunatic Asylums*, p. 215.

40 Parkes, *Fifty Years in the Making of Australian History*, p. 168.

41 'Death of Dr F N Manning'.

42 See Janette Pelosi, *Gladesville Mental Hospital Records and Their Uses for Family History* (unpublished thesis, Sydney, 1997).

43 Frederic Norton Manning, *Medical Certificates of Insanity* (Sydney: Government Printer, 1891), pp. 1–2.

44 Manning, *1882 Annual Report of the Inspector General of the Insane.*

45 Manning, *1886 Annual Report of the Inspector General of the Insane* (Sydney: Government Printer, 1887).

46 Manning, *Medical Certificates of Insanity*, pp. 4–5.

47 'Death of Dr F N Manning'.

48 Ibid.

49 'The Royal Commission on Hospitals for the Insane', *Argus*, 1 May 1886.

50 Manning, *Report on Lunatic Asylums*, p. 164.

51 Manning, *Report on Lunatic Asylums*, p. 155.

52 Ibid., pp. 160–1.

53 Ibid., p. 162.

54 Ibid., p. 165.

55 Ibid., p. 165.

56 Bonnie Davidson and Rosaleen Tidswell, 'Callan Park and John Gordon', *Peninsular Observer*, Vol. 37 (4), August 2002, p. 1.

57 Advertisement for Richardson and Wrench, *Sydney Morning Herald*, 6 December 1873.

58 For example, *NSW Legislative Assembly* transcript, 26 October 1893.

59 SRANSW, NRS 906, *Colonial Secretary Special Bundles: Erection of Callan Park Lunatic Asylum, 1873–79* [4/818.3].

3. The Kirkbride Complex

1 *Argus,* 20 January 1854.

2 Frederick Legard, 'The Railway Aspect', *The Age,* 10 June 1858.

3 TNA, [DG 9/264] 'Conveyance'.

4 TNA, [DG 9/266] 'Conveyance'.

5 Advertisement for the Victorian Collegiate Institution, *Argus,* 1 January 1864.

6 Advertisement for Mademoiselle Naegueli's Boarding and Day School, *Sydney Morning Herald,* 20 July 1867.

7 'A Modern Madhouse. Callan Park and its Inmates: Its Management and Methods', *Sunday Times,* 25 August 1895.

8 Manning, *1884 Annual Report of the Inspector General of the Insane* (Sydney: Government Printer, 1885).

9 'A Month in Kew Asylum and Yarra Bend', *Argus,* 22 July 1876.

10 Manning, *Report on Lunatic Asylums*, p. 212.

11 Manning, *1883 Annual Report of the Inspector General of the Insane.*

12 W. Lauder Lindsay, 'The Protection Bed and Its Uses', *American Journal of Insanity,* Vol. 36, 1879–80, p. 406.

13 'Laying of Memorial Stone at Callan Park', *Sydney Morning Herald,* 23 April 1883.

14 See Peta Longhurst, *The Foundations of Madness: the Role of the Built Environment in the Mental Institutions of New South Wales*, Sydney University: 2011, p. 86.

15 Manning, *Report on Lunatic Asylums*, p. 174.

16 'The Callan Park Asylum', *Sydney Morning Herald,* 26 August 1879.

17 Summary of 'Report' published in *Sydney Morning Herald,* 23 April 1877.

18 'Callan Park Asylum', *Sydney Morning Herald,* 16 June 1885.

19 'Insanity in New South Wales', *Sydney Morning Herald,* 20 June 1884.

20 'Laying of Memorial Stone at Callan Park'.

21 'Callan Park Asylum'.

22 'The Callan Park Lunatic Asylum', *Illustrated Sydney News,* 24 October 1885.

23 Manning, *1884 Annual Report of the Inspector General of the Insane.*

24 Ibid.

25 Ibid.

26 'Callan Park'.

27 *NSW Legislative Assembly* transcript, 22 September 1886.

28 'The Callan Park Asylum'.

29 Manning, *Report on Lunatic Asylums*, p. 175.

30 'A Modern Madhouse'.

31 Manning, *1888 Annual Report of the Inspector General of the Insane* (Sydney: Government Printer, 1889).

32 'Callan Park. A Great State Institution', *Sydney Mail,* 12 August 1903; photographs by Alfred Small, [Photographs of Callan Park Mental Hospital, 1903], Call Number [PX*D 241], State Library New South Wales.

33 See various *Annual Report of the Inspector General of the Insane.*

34 Manning, *Report on Lunatic Asylums*, p. 188.

35 'The Callan Park Asylum'.

36 Manning, *Report on Lunatic Asylums*, pp. 180–2, 188–9.

37 Manning, *1884 Annual Report of the Inspector General of the Insane.*

38 Manning, *1888 Annual Report of the Inspector General of the Insane.*

39 'The Callan Park Asylum'.

40 'A Modern Madhouse'.

41 Manning, *Report on Lunatic Asylums*, pp. 181–2.

42 'The Callan Park Asylum'.

43 *NSW Legislative Assembly* transcript, 23 February 1892.

44 'The Callan Park Asylum'.

45 Manning, *Report on Lunatic Asylums*, pp. 177–8.

46 Mary de Young, *Encyclopedia of Asylum Therapeutics, 1750–1950s* (North Carolina: McFarland & Company, Inc, 2015), p. 187, summarising Thomas Power, *Report on the effects of the Turkish bath in the treatment of insanity, for the Board of Governors*, Cork: 1865.

47 Manning, *1890 Annual Report of the Inspector General of the Insane* (Sydney: Government Printer, 1891).

48 Manning, *1886 Annual Report of the Inspector General of the Insane.*

49 'A Modern Madhouse'.

50 de Young, *Encyclopedia of Asylum Therapeutics*, pp. 195–6.

51 'Callan Park Asylum'.

52 'A Modern Madhouse'.

53 'Callan Park Asylum'.

54 Manning, *1885 Annual Report of the Inspector General of the Insane.*

55 Manning, *1886 Annual Report of the Inspector General of the Insane.*

56 'A Modern Madhouse'.

57 Manning, *1885 Annual Report of the Inspector General of the Insane.*

58 'Ball at Callan Park Asylum', *Balmain Observer and Western Suburbs Advertiser,* 25 August 1888.

59 Manning, *1886 Annual Report of the Inspector General of the Insane.*

60 Manning, *1889 Annual Report of the Inspector General of the Insane* (Sydney: Government Printer, 1890).

61 Manning, *Report on Lunatic Asylums*, p. 195.

62 'The Callan Park Asylum'.

63 Manning, *1891 Annual Report of the Inspector General of the Insane* (Sydney: Government Printer, 1892).

64 'Callan Park Asylum'.

65 Ibid.

66 'The Callan Park Lunatic Asylum'.

67 Manning, *The Causation and Prevention of Insanity*, p. 9.

68 'The Callan Park Asylum'.

69 'A Modern Madhouse'.

70 Manning, *1888 Annual Report of the Inspector General of the Insane.*

71 Manning, *1884 Annual Report of the Inspector General of the Insane.*

72 Manning, *1892 Annual Report of the Inspector General of the Insane.*

73 'A Modern Madhouse'. The patient was possibly John Cane, who was an engineer. Cane was resident at Gladesville from 1872, and then Callan Park from September 1879 when he was transferred there. He was discharged in 1880 as cured of his dementia.

74 Manning, *1887 Annual Report of the Inspector General of the Insane* (Sydney: Government Printer, 1888).

75 Manning, *1889 Annual Report of the Inspector General of the Insane.*

76 Ibid.

77 Ibid.

78 'The Callan Park Asylum'.

79 Manning, *1888 Annual Report of the Inspector General of the Insane.*

80 Manning, *Report on Lunatic Asylums*, p. 156.

81 Manning, *Address in Psychological Medicine*, p. 12.

82 Ibid.

83 Garton, *Medicine and Madness*, p. 109.

84 Manning, *1887 Annual Report of the Inspector General of the Insane.*

85 Manning, *1888 Annual Report of the Inspector General of the Insane.*

86 Manning, *1889 Annual Report of the Inspector General of the Insane.*

87 Garton, *Medicine and Madness*, p. 109.

88 *NSW Legislative Assembly* transcript, 20 September 1887.

89 Garton, *Medicine and Madness*, p. 109.

90 Pasquin, 'The Social Kaleidoscope'.

91 *NSW Legislative Assembly* transcript, 22 May 1894.

92 Ibid.

93 Manning, *1890 Annual Report of the Inspector General of the Insane.*

94 Manning, *1887 Annual Report of the Inspector General of the Insane.*

95 Ibid.

96 Manning, *1884 Annual Report of the Inspector General of the Insane.*

4. Attendants and the Routine

1 Garton, *Medicine and Madness,* p. 168.

2 Manning, 1887 *Annual Report of the Inspector General of the Insane.*

3 *NSW Legislative Assembly* transcript, 10 November 1897.

4 Manning, *Report on Lunatic Asylums,* p. 156.

5 *NSW Legislative Assembly* transcript, 20 November 1884.

6 'Death of Dr F N Manning'.

7 'Dr Chisholm Ross', *Goulburn Evening Penny Post,* 5 September 1903.

8 'Civil Service List' published in the *Sydney Morning Herald,* 1 May 1885.

9 See relevant *Civil Service Lists* for each year.

10 Manning, *1885 Annual Report of the Inspector General of the Insane.*

11 Manning, *1886 Annual Report of the Inspector General of the Insane.*

12 Ibid.

13 Ibid.

14 *Sydney Morning Herald,* 2 March 1891.

15 'Vegetable Gardening', *Cumberland Argus and Fruitgrowers Advocate,* 19 March 1898.

16 Advertisement in many newspapers and at different times; for example: *Manning River Times and Advocate for the Northern Coast Districts of New South Wales,* 11 February 1899.

17 *NSW Legislative Assembly* transcript, 23 April 1884.

18 *NSW Legislative Assembly* transcript, 23 February 1892.

19 Manning, *Report on Lunatic Asylums,* p. 167.

20 Manning, *1885 Annual Report of the Inspector General of the Insane.*

21 *NSW Legislative Assembly* transcript, 23 June 1886.

22 Manning, *1889 Annual Report of the Inspector General of the Insane.*

23 Manning, *1891 Annual Report of the Inspector General of the Insane.*

24 *NSW Legislative Assembly* transcript, 2 February 1892.

25 Ibid.

26 *NSW Legislative Assembly* transcript, 1 November 1892.

27 *NSW Legislative Assembly* transcript, 23 February 1892.

28 Ibid.

29 'Callan Park Asylum'.

30 Ibid.

31 Sources for Arthur Brown, unless otherwise cited, are: SRANSW, NRS 4994, *Callan Park Medical Case Book* [3/4652A] and NRS 4998, *Callan Park Medical Journal* [3/7045].

32 SRANSW, NRS 4998, *Callan Park Medical Journal* [3/7045].

33 Vagabond, the man who posed as an attendant in Kew and Yarra Bend in Melbourne, described such a situation ('A Month in Kew Asylum and Yarra Bend', *Argus,* 22 July 1876). While supervising an aggressive patient who had already

been restrained, Vagabond was assaulted with a punch to the eye and scratched his finger, which became infected. Despite his pain, Vagabond described staying with the patient to ensure he did not hurt himself. He finished the recount with the mild reminder that, 'All these little accidents are what an attendant must expect'.

34 SRANSW, NRS 4998, *Callan Park Medical Journal* [3/7045].

35 Ibid.

36 Ibid.

37 Ibid.

38 Ibid.

39 Ibid.

40 'Callan Park Asylum'.

41 *NSW Legislative Assembly* transcript, 23 February 1892.

42 Ibid.

43 These were recorded in SRANSW, NRS 4998, *Callan Park Medical Journal* [3/7045].

44 'A Remarkable Case, An Escapee from Callan Park', *Cumberland Argus and Fruitgrowers Advocate,* 6 August 1898.

45 SRANSW, NRS 4998, *Callan Park Medical Journal* [3/7045].

46 Ibid.

47 Ibid.

48 Ibid.

49 Ibid.

50 Warnings were recorded in SRANSW, NRS 4998, *Callan Park Medical Journal* [3/7045].

51 Fines were recorded in Ibid.

52 *NSW Legislative Assembly* transcript, 15 February 1892.

53 'Inquiry about Miss M. A. Fairbairn', *Sydney Morning Herald,* 26 July 1900.

54 *NSW Legislative Assembly* transcript, 16 August 1900.

55 *NSW Legislative Assembly* transcript, 23 August 1900.

56 'Intercolonial News', *Newcastle Morning Herald and Miners' Advocate,* 20 August 1900.

57 'The Callan Park Inquiry', *Wagga Wagga Express,* 31 July 1900.

58 *NSW Legislative Assembly* transcript, 4 October 1900.

59 'Mr E. M. Betts', *Sydney Morning Herald,* 24 January 1902.

60 *NSW Legislative Assembly* transcript, 19 October 1900.

61 'The Asylum Changes', *Cumberland Argus and Fruitgrowers Advocate,* 10 October 1900.

62 'Obituary', *Sydney Morning Herald,* 8 October 1934.

63 Ibid.

64 'The Late Dr Chisholm Ross', *Glen Innes Examiner,* 9 October 1934.

65 'Dr Chisholm Ross', *Goulburn Evening Penny Post,* 5 September 1903.

66 'The Late Dr Blaxland', *Sydney Mail,* 27 April 1904.

67 Ibid.

68 'In Memoriam', *Sydney Morning Herald,* 10 April 1905.

5. The Admission Process

1 This was discussed in conjunction with the case of a lunatic named Edward William Easwell in *NSW Legislative Assembly* transcript 12 November 1895.

2 Manning, *1887 Annual Report of the Inspector General of the Insane.*

3 'Water Police Court', *Empire,* 12 May 1869.

4 'Darlinghurst Gaol', *Freeman's Journal,* 25 July 1874.

5 SRANSW, NRS 2523, *Sydney Gaol Description Book,* 1869, Reel 857.

6 Darlinghurst Gaol was equipped with padded cells for criminal lunatics ('Darlinghurst Gaol'), but there is no evidence that Legard was incarcerated in one of these.

7 Arthur Holroyd, 'Department of the Master in Lunacy', *Sydney Morning Herald,* 3 May 1881.

8 Frederic Norton Manning, 'Report for 1873 on the Gladesville Hospital for the Insane', *Clarence and Richmond Examiner and New England Advertiser,* 12 May 1874.

9 For this information I am greatly indebted to Bob Taylor and Brian Woodlands.

10 For William Andrew's patient records see SRANSW, NRS 4994, *Callan Park Medical Case Book* [3/4652].

6. Men Very Far from Home

1 13 November 1888.

2 Sources for Fillipo Parcelli are, unless otherwise cited, SRANSW, NRS 5019, *Reception House Medical Case Book* [11/2153]; NRS 5031, *Gladesville Medical Case Book* [4/8164 and 4/8171]; NRS 5047, *Gladesville Addresses of Patients' Friends* [4/10565]; NRS 4994, *Callan Park Medical Case Book* [3/4652]; NRS 4998, *Callan Park Medical Journal* [3/7045]; NRS 2602, *Young Gaol Entrance Book* [6/5439]; NRS 2604, *Young Gaol Description Book* [6/5436].

3 Manning, *The Causation and Prevention of Insanity,* p. 2.

4 SRANSW, NRS 2613, *Young Gaol Punishment Book* [7/13499].

5 Source for William Clancy is, unless otherwise cited, SRANSW, NRS 4994, *Callan Park Medical Case Book* [3/4652].

6 Manning, *Address in Psychological Medicine,* p. 19.

7 *NSW Legislative Assembly* transcript, 22 September 1886.

8 *NSW Legislative Assembly* transcript, 23 February 1892.

9 Manning, *1881 Annual Report of the Inspector General of the Insane.*

10 Manning, *1883 Annual Report of the Inspector General of the Insane.*

11 Frederic Norton Manning, 'The Hospitals for the Insane', *Sydney Morning Herald,* 3 May 1886.

12 Derrick I. Stone and Sue Mackinnon, *Life on the Australian Goldfields* (Frenchs Forest: Reed, 1982), p. 8.

13 'Bathurst', *Sydney Morning Herald,* 16 May 1851.

14 'Chinese Riot at Bathurst', *Evening News,* 17 July 1877.

15 Sources for Chan Long, Ah Chun and Ah Fuun are, unless otherwise cited, SRANSW, NRS 5031, *Gladesville Medical Case Books* [4/8162, 4/8164 and 4/8165]; NRS 4994, *Callan Park Medical Case Book* [3/4652]; NRS 4998, *Callan Park Medical Journal* [3/7045].

16 Manning, *The Causation and Prevention of Insanity,* p. 7.

17 *NSW Legislative Assembly* transcript, 23 April 1884.

18 Pasquin, 'The Social Kaleidoscope'.

19 Manning, 'The Hospitals for the Insane'.

20 Sources for Khumis Baroot and James Wilson Ellis, unless otherwise cited, are: SRANSW, NRS 4994, *Callan Park Medical Case Book* [3/4652]; NRS 4998, *Callan Park Medical Journal* [3/7045].

7. George Morton

1 Sources for Arthur O'Connor (alias George Morton), unless otherwise cited, are: SRANSW, NRS 5019, *Reception House Medical Case Book* [11/2154]; NRS 4994, *Callan Park Medical Case Book* [3/4652A]; NRS 4998, *Callan Park Medical Journal* [3/7045]; NRS 5001, *Callan Park Correspondence from Patients* [3/4921]; TNA, [HO 144/3/10963] 'Home Office File for Arthur O'Connor'.

2 Thomas Cooper, 'The Lion of Freedom', *Northern Star and Leeds General Advertiser,* 11 September 1841.

3 'Great Britain. O'Connor and John Brown in Court', *Freeman's Journal,* 11 May 1872.

4 Tuke ran the Manor House Asylum in Chiswick, in England, and promoted the use of non-restraint methods of treatment and control in asylums.

5 The Fenians were a radical group dedicated to the establishment of an independent Irish Republic. In England, their exploits were often violent.

6 TNA, HO 10963/28.

7 'Great Britain. O'Connor and John Brown in Court'.

8 'Attack on Her Majesty', *Adelaide Observer,* 13 April 1872.

9 TNA, HO 10963/28.

10 'The Document Presented by O'Connor to the Queen for her Signature', *Launceston Examiner,* 1 June 1872.

11 'Great Britain. O'Connor and John Brown in Court'.

12 Ibid.

13 'Trial of O'Connor for Pointing a Pistol at the Queen', *The Age,* 1 June 1872.

14 Ibid.

15 TNA, HO 10963/5.

16 TNA, HO 10963/8.

17 TNA, HO 10963/9.

18 Ibid.

19 TNA, HO 10963/10.

20 Ibid.

21 TNA, HO 10963/19.

22 TNA, HO 10963/13.

23 TNA, HO 10963/17.

24 TNA, HO 10963/20.

25 The advertisement likely responded to read: 'Wanted, a single man, as assistant butcher; must be a good scholar' (*Maitland Mercury and Hunter River General Advertiser,* 2 January 1873) or perhaps 'Wanted, a shopman; to make himself otherwise useful. Wages liberal to sober man' (*Maitland Mercury and Hunter River General Advertiser,* 22 April 1873).

26 TNA, HO 10963/20.

27 TNA, HO 10963/22.

28 'Morpeth', *Evening News,* 25 February 1884.

29 Henry Geary's advertisement to replace him: 'Wanted, a Butcher to Slaughter and make himself useful, must be a scholar', *Maitland Mercury and Hunter River General Advertiser,* 30 September 1873.

30 TNA, HO 10963/21.

31 TNA, HO 10963/22.

32 TNA, HO 10963/22.

33 TNA, HO 10963/23.

34 TNA, HO 10963/24.

35 TNA, HO 10963/26.

36 Ibid.

37 TNA, HO 10963/25.

38 TNA, HO 10963/26.

39 Ibid.

40 TNA, HO 10963/28.

41 Ibid.

42 Ibid.

43 Ibid.

44 Ibid.

45 Ibid.

46 TNA, HO 10963/28a.

47 TNA, HO 10963/30.

48 TNA, HO 10963/32.

49 TNA, HO 10963/34.

50 TNA, HO 10963/33.
51 TNA, HO 10963/34.
52 SRANSW, NRS 5593, *Inspector General of the Insane Register of Admissions* [3/7064].
53 TNA, HO 10963/35.
54 TNA, HO 10963/37.
55 TNA, HO 10963/38; 10963/39.
56 Manning, *1886 Annual Report of the Inspector General of the Insane.*
57 *An Act to consolidate and amend the Law relating to the Insane* [4th February, 1879], Part IX (183).
58 Manning, *Report on Lunatic Asylums*, p. 190.
59 TNA, HO 10963/40.

8.Samuel Payne

1 All information on Samuel Payne, unless otherwise cited, comes from SRANSW, NRS 5031, *Gladesville Medical Case Book* [4/8162]; NRS 5042, *Gladesville Warrants* [8/2355]; NRS 4994, *Callan Park Medical Case Book* [3/4652]; NRS 4998, *Callan Park Medical Journal* [3/7045].
2 'Sullivan, the New Zealand Murderer. Discharge of the Prisoner', *Bendigo Advertiser,* 1 May 1876.
3 'Sullivan the Murderer', *Evening News,* 1 May 1876.
4 The narrative of the Burgess gang comes from Steve Watters (Ministry for Culture and Heritage), 'Maungatapu Murders, 1866', www.nzhistory.net.nz/culture/further-sources-maungatapu-murders, updated 17 September 2015 (accessed 4 October 2016).
5 Superintendent Alfred Saunders argued that Sullivan was entitled to a free pardon (Archives New Zealand, Te Rua Mahara o te Kawanatanga [Christchurch Regional Office], *Inwards Correspondence Provincial Secretary,* Canterbury Provincial Archives [CAAR, CH287, CP85, ICPS 1966/1866]).
6 'Sullivan the Murderer'.
7 *Sydney Morning Herald,* 8 May 1876.
8 'The Murderer Sullivan', *Wagga Wagga Advertiser,* 17 May 1876.
9 'Reported Visit to Sydney of Sullivan the Murderer', *Evening News,* 10 September 1877.
10 'The Murderer Sullivan', *Evening News,* 2 October 1877.

9. Escapees

1 Examples from this chapter have been taken from: SRANSW, NRS 4994, *Callan Park Medical Case Book* [3/4652]; NRS 4998, *Callan Park Medical Journal* [3/7045]; particularly relevant patients' records have been explicitly referenced below.
2 'Callan Park Asylum'.
3 Manning, *Report on Lunatic Asylums*, p. 210.

4 Manning, *1881 Annual Report of the Inspector General of the Insane.*

5 In addition to the sources listed at the beginning of this chapter, Sipple is also recorded in: SRANSW, NRS 5031, *Gladesville Medical Case Book* [4/8159].

6 In addition to the sources listed at the beginning of this chapter, Clubb is also recorded in: SRANSW, NRS 5019, *Reception House Medical Case Book* [11/2153]; SRANSW, NRS 5031, *Gladesville Medical Case Book* [4/8165]; NRS 5047, *Gladesville Addresses of Patients' Friends* [4/10565]; NRS 4984, *Callan Park Case Papers* [3/3317].

7 'Escaped Lunatic', *NSW Police Gazette,* 11 October 1882.

8 *NSW Police Gazette,* 18 October 1882.

9 In addition to the sources listed at the beginning of this chapter, Swain is also recorded in: SRANSW, NRS 5031, *Gladesville Medical Case Book* [4/8172].

10. Voluntary Admissions

1 Sources for William Dwyer, unless otherwise cited, are: SRANSW, NRS 5019, *Reception House Medical Case Book* [11/2154]; NRS 4994, *Callan Park Medical Case Books* [3/4652, 3/4652A]; NRS 4998, *Callan Park Medical Journals* [3/7045, 3/7046].

2 Though where exactly this house was is unclear. There were various cottages scattered over Callan Park, but where the medical superintendent lived pre-Kirkbride is not documented. The cottages on Manning Road are a likely possibility indicated by Dwyer's easy escape, but their distance from Garryowen suggests perhaps another location.

3 A 'glazier's diamond' was a tool used for cutting or marking glass. In 1879 such a tool was valued at £1 1s and was regarded as something worth stealing (as recounted in a different case in 'Milicent Police Court', *Border Watch,* 8 February 1879).

4 Manning, *1881 Annual Report of the Inspector General of the Insane.*

5 Sources for Charles Merritt, unless otherwise cited, are: SRANSW, NRS 4994, *Callan Park Medical Case Book* [3/4652]; NRS 4998, *Callan Park Medical Journal* [3/7045]; NRS 5113, *Parramatta Medical Case Book* [6/5371].

6 Sources for William Andrews, unless otherwise cited, are: SRANSW, NRS 4994, *Callan Park Medical Case Book* [3/4652]; NRS 4998, *Callan Park Medical Journal* [3/7045].

7 Sources for George Merry, unless otherwise cited, are: SRANSW, NRS 5019, *Reception House Medical Case Book* [11/2153]; NRS 4994, *Callan Park Medical Case Book* [3/4652]; NRS 4998, *Callan Park Medical Journal* [3/7045]; NRS 13340 *Deceased Estate Files – File for George Merry date duty paid 29/7/1896* [20/65B].

8 'Missing Friends', *NSW Police Gazette,* 12 February 1873.

9 'In the estate of George Merry, late of Sydney, in the Colony of New South Wales, gold-miner, deceased', *Government Gazette,* 1 October 1896.

10 Sources for Samuel Wade, unless otherwise cited, are: SRANSW, NRS 5019, *Reception House Medical Case Book* [11/2153]; NRS5047, *Gladesville Addresses of Patients' Friends* [4/10565]; NRS 4994, *Callan Park Medical Case Book* [3/4652]; NRS 4998, *Callan Park Medical Journal* [3/7045].

11. Recovered

1 Manning, *Report on Lunatic Asylums*, pp. 154–5.

2 Sources for Joshua Fitzpatrick, unless otherwise cited, are: SRANSW, NRS 5019, *Reception House Medical Case Book* [11/2153]; NRS 5031, *Gladesville Medical Case Book* [4/8162]; NRS 5043, *Gladesville Medical Journal* [8/2326B]; NRS 4994, *Callan Park Medical Case Book* [3/4652]; NRS 4998, *Callan Park Medical Journal* [3/7045]; NRS 5113, *Parramatta Medical Case Book* [6/5357].

3 'Missing Friends', *NSW Police Gazette*, 5 December 1877.

4 Ibid.

5 'Escaped Lunatic', *NSW Police Gazette*, 14 July 1880.

6 Sources for James McMahon, unless otherwise cited, are: SRANSW, NRS 5019, *Reception House Medical Case Book* [11/2153]; NRS 4994, *Callan Park Medical Case Book* [3/4652]; NRS 4998, *Callan Park Medical Journal* [3/7045].

7 Manning, *Report on Lunatic Asylums*, p. 154.

8 Ibid.

9 Sources for Henry Jones, unless otherwise cited, are: SRANSW, NRS 4994, *Callan Park Medical Case Book* [3/4652]; NRS 4998, *Callan Park Medical Journal* [3/7045].

12. Chronic Patients

1 Manning, *1881 Annual Report of the Inspector General of the Insane*.

2 Manning, *1883 Annual Report of the Inspector General of the Insane*.

3 Source for Josias Keenan, unless otherwise cited, is: SRANSW, NRS 4994, *Callan Park Medical Case Book* [3/4652].

4 'Dr. John McDonald Brennan', *Catholic Press*, 20 May 1909.

5 Sources for William Brennan, unless otherwise cited, are: SRANSW, NRS 5019, *Reception House Medical Case Book* [11/2153]; NRS 4994, *Callan Park Medical Case Books* [3/4652, 3/4652A]; NRS 4998, *Callan Park Medical Journal* [3/7045].

6 'Dr John McDonald Brennan'.

7 SRANSW, NRS 5001, *Callan Park Correspondence from Patients* [3/4921].

8 Sources for Terence McGuire, unless otherwise cited, are: SRANSW, NRS 4994, *Callan Park Medical Case Book* [3/4652]; NRS 4998, *Callan Park Medical Journal* [3/7045].

9 Sources for Simon Patrick Holland, unless otherwise cited, are: SRANSW, NRS 5019, *Reception House Medical Case Book* [11/2153]; NRS 5031, *Gladesville Medical Case Book* [4/8160]; NRS 4994, *Callan Park Medical Case Book* [3/4652]; NRS 4998, *Callan Park Medical Journal* [3/7045].

10 Manning, *The Causation and Prevention of Insanity*, p. 10.

11 Manning, *Address in Psychological Medicine*, p. 14.

12 Manning, 'The Hospitals for the Insane'.

13 'Dr John McDonald Brennan'.

14 Advertisement 'Dr J M Brennan' occurred in the *Balmain Observer and Western Suburbs Advertiser* on multiple dates including: 1 October 1904, 7 January 1905,

18 March 1905.

15 Sources for Jeremiah Lynch, unless otherwise cited, are: SRANSW, NRS 5019, *Reception House Medical Case Book* [11/2153]; NRS 4994, *Callan Park Medical Case Book* [3/4652)]; NRS 4998, *Callan Park Medical Journal* [3/7045]; NRS 4946, *Liverpool Asylum Registers of Admissions and Discharges 1895* [7/5308], Reel 1399.

16 'Deserters from Her Majesty's Service', *NSW Police Gazette,* 18 July 1877, p. 234.

17 'Offences not otherwise described', *NSW Police Gazette,* 5 March 1879, p. 94.

18 'Insolvent Proceedings', *The Maitland Mercury and Hunter River General Advertiser,* 24 July 1886.

19 Manning, *1887 Annual Report of the Inspector General of the Insane.*

20 Sources for James Daniel Webster, unless otherwise cited, are: SRANSW, NRS 5019, *Reception House Medical Case Book* [11/2153]; NRS 4994, *Callan Park Medical Case Book* [3/4652]; NRS 12252 and 12253, *Master in Lunacy Maintenance Ledgers* and *Books* [3/14224–7, 3/14229].

21 Manning, *1890 Annual Report of the Inspector General of the Insane.*

22 Manning, *1891 Annual Report of the Inspector General of the Insane.*

23 *NSW Legislative Assembly* transcript, 23 February 1892.

24 Source for Samuel Bennett, unless otherwise cited, is: SRANSW, NRS 4994, *Callan Park Medical Case Book* [3/4652].

25 Sources for Henry Robert Black, unless otherwise cited, are: SRANSW, NRS 4994, *Callan Park Medical Case Book* [3/4652]; NRS 4998, *Callan Park Medical Journal* [3/7045].

26 Sources for John Burton Cox, unless otherwise cited, are: SRANSW, NRS 5019, *Reception House Medical Case Book* [11/2154]; NRS 4994, *Callan Park Medical Case Book* [3/4652A]; NRS 4998, *Callan Park Medical Journal* [3/7045].

27 Sources for Thomas Manning, unless otherwise cited, are: SRANSW, NRS 5019, *Reception House Medical Case Book* [11/2152]; NRS 4994, *Callan Park Medical Case Book* [3/4652].

28 *NSW Legislative Assembly* transcript, 1 February 1894.

29 Sources for John Evans, unless otherwise cited, are: SRANSW, NRS 4994, *Callan Park Medical Case Book* [3/4652]; NRS 4984, *Callan Park Case Papers 1878–1882* [3/3317].

Epilogue

1 Manning, *1879 Annual Report of the Inspector General of the Insane* (Sydney: Government Printer, 1880) and *1881 Annual Report of the Inspector General of the Insane.*

BIBLIOGRAPHY

NEWSPAPERS AND PERIODICALS

Adelaide Observer
The Age
Argus
Australian Town and Country Journal
Balmain Observer and Western Suburbs Advertiser
Bendigo Advertiser
Border Watch
Canberra Times
Catholic Press
Clarence and Richmond Examiner and New England Advertiser
Cumberland Argus and Fruitgrowers Advocate
Daily Telegraph
Empire
Evening News
Freeman's Journal
Glen Innes Examiner
Goulburn Evening Penny Post
Government Gazette
Herald Sun
Illustrated Sydney News
Launceston Examiner
Maitland Mercury and Hunter River General Advertiser
Manning River Times and Advocate for the Northern Coast Districts of New South Wales
Newcastle Morning Herald and Miners' Advocate
Newcastle Sun
Northern Star and Leeds General Advertiser
NSW Police Gazette
Sunday Times

Sydney Mail
Sydney Mail and New South Wales Advertiser
Sydney Morning Herald
Wagga Wagga Express
Weekly Times

ARCHIVAL SOURCES

Borthwick Institute for Archives, University of York

Institution Act Book [INST/AB/20]
Ordination papers [ORD/P/1839] and [ORD/D/1840]
Cecilia Legard of Bramham (Prog), February 1855

East Riding Archives

Insanity of Thomas and William Legard [DDGR/43/17/12]
Thomas Legard placed in madhouse [DDGR/43/17/24]
Registers of Ganton 1846–1852

The National Archives UK

[C 211/15/L90] 'Sir Thomas Legard, bart of Ganton, Yorkshire: commission and inquisition of lunacy, into his state of mind and his property'
[DG 9/264] 'Conveyance'
[DG 9/266] 'Conveyance'
[HO 107] 'Census Returns' (1851)
[HO 144/3/10963] 'Home Office File for Arthur O'Connor'
[MH 94/1-47] 'UK Lunacy Patients Admission Registers, 1846–1912'

State Archives and Records Authority of New South Wales

NRS 906 *Colonial Secretary Special Bundles: Erection of Callan Park Lunatic Asylum, 1873–79* [4/818.3]
NRS 2523 *Sydney Gaol Description Book, 1869*, Reel 857
NRS 2602 *Young Gaol Entrance Book* [6/5439]
NRS 2604 *Young Gaol Description Book* [6/5436]
NRS 2613 *Young Gaol Punishment Book* [7/13499]

NRS 4946 *Liverpool Asylum Registers of Admissions and Discharges 1895* [7/5308], Reel 1399
NRS 4984, *Callan Park Case Papers 1878–82* [3/3317]
NRS 4994, *Callan Park Medical Case Books* [3/4651-52A]
NRS 4998, *Callan Park Medical Journals* [3/7045-47]
NRS 5001, *Callan Park Letters from Patients, 1881-1919* [3/4921] – patient George Morton
NRS 5019 *Darlinghurst Reception House Medical Case Books* [11/2152-54]
NRS 5031 *Gladesville Medical Case Books* [4/8149, 4/8153, 4/8155, 4/8155-65, 4/8171-72 and 4/8198]
NRS 5042 *Gladesville Warrants of Admission 1863–79* [8/2350 and 8/2355]
NRS 5043 *Gladesville Medical Journal* [8/2326B]
NRS 5047 *Gladesville Register of Addresses of Patients' Friends, 1874–80* [4/10565]
NRS 5059 *Gladesville Miscellaneous Papers c.1855–99* [4/8136.2]
NRS 5066 *Newcastle Medical Case Book* [34/3483]
NRS 5113 *Parramatta Medical Case Books* [6/5357, 6/5371]
NRS 5593 *Inspector General of Mental Hospitals Patient's Admission Register (males)* [3/7064]
NRS 12252 *Maintenance Books, 1879–84* [3/14224-26]
NRS 12253 *Maintenance Ledgers* [3/14227,3/14229]
NRS 13340 *Deceased Estate Files – File for George Merry date duty paid 29/7/1896* [20/65B]

Other

An Act to consolidate and amend the Law relating to the Insane [4 February 1879]
Archives New Zealand, Te Rua Mahara o te Kawanatanga [Christchurch Regional Office], *Inwards Correspondence Provincial Secretary*, Canterbury Provincial Archives [CAAR, CH287, CP85, ICPS 1966/1866] viewed at 'The remission of Sullivan – Maungatapu murders', https://nzhistory.govt.nz/media/interactive/the-remission-of-sullivan-letter, (Ministry for Culture and Heritage), updated 13 August 2015
Balmain Directory
Charterhouse School Archive, *Alumni Carthusiani*
Charterhouse School Archive, *Charterhouse Register* 1769–1872
NSW Legislative Assembly Votes and Proceedings

New Zealand Electoral Roll (1890)
Victorian Hansard
Victorian Legislative Assembly, *Reports*

BOOKS AND ARTICLES

Beckett, Ray and Richard, *Hangman: The Life and Times of Alexander Green Public Executioner to the Colony of New South Wales*, Melbourne: Nelson, 1980

Bronte, C, *Jane Eyre, An Autobiography*, London: Service & Paton, 1897

Davidson, Bonnie and Tidswell, Rosaleen, 'Callan Park and John Gordon', *Peninsular Observer*, Vol. 37 (4), August 2002, p. 1

Garton, Stephen, *Medicine and Madness. A Social History of Insanity in NSW 1880–1940,* Kensington: New South Wales University Press, 1988

Legard, James Digby, *The Legards of Anlaby & Ganton: Their Neighbours & Neighbourhood,* London: Simpkin, Marshall, Hamilton, Kent & Co., 1926

Lindsay, W Lauder, 'The Protection Bed and Its Uses', *American Journal of Insanity*, Vol. 36, 1879–80, pp. 404–21

Manning, Frederic Norton, *Address Delivered on Resigning Charge as Medical Superintendent of the Hospitals for the Insane at Gladesville and Callan Park*, Sydney: Gibbs, Shallard, & Co, 1879

Manning, F N, *Address in Psychological Medicine*, Sydney: Government Printer, 1888

Manning, F N, *Medical Certificates of Insanity*, Sydney: Government Printer, 1891

Manning, F N, *Report of the Inspector General of the Insane,* Sydney: Government Printer, 1879–1898

Manning, F N, *Report on Lunatic Asylums*, Sydney: Government Printer, 1868

Manning, F N, *The Causation and Prevention of Insanity*, Sydney: Government Printer, 1880

Parkes, Henry, *Fifty Years in the Making of Australian History*, North Carolina: Hayes Barton Press, 2006

Perceval, J, *A Narrative of the treatment experienced by a gentleman during a state of mental derangement; designed to explain the causes and the nature of insanity, and to expose the injudicious conduct pursued towards many unfortunate sufferers under that calamity*, London: Effingham Wilson, 1840

Reade, C, *Hard Cash, A Matter-of-Fact Romance*, London: Chatto and Windus, 1862

Stone, Derrick I and Mackinnon, Sue, *Life on the Australian Goldfields,* Frenchs Forest: Reed, 1982

Tod, A H, *Charterhouse*, London: George Bell and Sons, 1900

Trollope, Anthony (ed. John Morley), *Thackeray. English Men of Letters Series*, London: Macmillan, 1879

de Young, Mary, *Encyclopedia of Asylum Therapeutics, 1750–1950s*, North Carolina: McFarland & Company, Inc, 2015

UNPUBLISHED THESES

Longhurst, Peta, *The Foundations of Madness: the Role of the Built Environment in the Mental Institutions of New South Wales*, unpublished thesis, Sydney University, 2011

Pelosi, Janette, *Gladesville Mental Hospital Records and Their Uses for Family History*, unpublished thesis, Sydney, 1997

WEBSITES

Caroline Simpson Library, http://museum.collection.hht.net.au/search.do;jsessionid=RW93HOtM3v2DiBZNm+WAqLQA?id=1133&db=object&page=1&view=detail, accessed 4 October 2016

Watters, Steve (Ministry for Culture and Heritage), 'Maungatapu Murders, 1866', www.nzhistory.net.nz/culture/further-sources-maungatapu-murders, updated 17 September 2015, accessed 4 October 2016

PHOTOGRAPH ALBUMS

Small, Alfred, [Photographs of Callan Park Mental Hospital, 1903], Call Number [PX*D 241], State Library New South Wales

Whitling, Arthur, [Family and holiday album, 1899–1908/ Arthur Whitling], Call Number [PXE 917], State Library New South Wales

INDEX

(*P*) indicates a patient at Callan Park; (*S*) indicates a member of Callan Park's staff. Numbers in italics refer to the plates

www.ingramcontent.com/pod-product-compliance
Ingram Content Group Australia Pty Ltd
76 Discovery Rd, Dandenong South VIC 3175, AU
AUHW020137130726
429791AU00003B/82

9 781925 588965